PEAK 40

Also by Dr Marc Bubbs

Peak: The New Science of Athletic Performance
That Is Revolutionizing Sports

PEAK 40

The New Science
of **Mid-Life Health** for
a Leaner, Stronger Body
and a Sharper Mind

Dr Marc Bubbs

ND, MSc, CISSN, CSCS

Chelsea Green Publishing
White River Junction, Vermont
London, UK

Project Manager: Patricia Stone
Developmental Editor: Muna Reyal
Copy Editor: Jo Roberts-Miller
Proofreader: Anne Sheasby
Indexer: Linda Hallinger
Designer: Melissa Jacobson

Printed in Canada.
First printing April 2021.
10 9 8 7 6 5 4 3 2 1   21 22 23 24 25

Our Commitment to Green Publishing

Chelsea Green sees publishing as a tool for cultural change and ecological stewardship. We strive to align our book manufacturing practices with our editorial mission and to reduce the impact of our business enterprise in the environment. We print our books and catalogs on chlorine-free recycled paper, using vegetable-based inks whenever possible. This book may cost slightly more because it was printed on paper that contains recycled fiber, and we hope you'll agree that it's worth it. *Peak 40* was printed on paper supplied by Marquis that is made of recycled materials and other controlled sources.

Library of Congress Cataloging-in-Publication Data
Names: Bubbs, Marc, author.
Title: Peak 40 : the new science of mid-life health for a leaner, stronger body and a sharper mind /
    Dr. Marc Bubbs, ND, MSc, CISSN, CSCS.
Other titles: Peak forty
Description: White River Junction : Chelsea Green Publishing, 2021. | Includes bibliographical
    references and index.
Identifiers: LCCN 2021010777 (print) | LCCN 2021010778 (ebook)
    | ISBN 9781645020738 (paperback) | ISBN 9781645020745 (ebook)
Subjects: LCSH: Physical fitness — Health aspects. | Exercise — Physiological aspects.
    | Nutrition. | Middle-age — Health aspects.
Classification: LCC RA781 .B824 2021 (print) | LCC RA781 (ebook) | DDC 613.7 – dc23
LC record available at https://lccn.loc.gov/2021010777
LC ebook record available at https://lccn.loc.gov/2021010778

Chelsea Green Publishing
85 North Main Street, Suite 120
White River Junction, Vermont USA

Somerset House
London, UK

www.chelseagreen.com

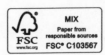

To my wife and three beautiful daughters
for all the love in the world.

To my mom, my dad and my sister
for all the support over the years.

To my good friend Andrew Svoboda,
whose talents never got to see mid life,
but whose influence continues.

CONTENTS

The Mid-Life U-Turn

A chieve success and happiness will follow. Get a good job, earn a good living and you'll be happy. Right? If happiness does indeed come *after* success, you would expect mid life to be the happiest time of most people's lives, a period traditionally marked by the pinnacle of achievement and career success, but here's the rub: happiness does not necessarily follow success.

In mid life, the alarming fact is that, despite what professional, material or personal success you may have achieved after years of effort and dedication, as well as the miracle of kids for many and/or a wide social network, research shows happiness dips to a lifetime low. How could this be? No matter if you drive a bus, run a company, play professional sport or head a Fortune 500 company, the relationship appears to hold true. For how long does this lull in happiness last? Apparently, the bottom of the U-shaped bell curve of happiness continues until the age of 48. (That's an awfully long time not to feel your happiest.)

It's Time to Be More, Not Do More

In mid life, it's easy for the years of hard work, lack of sleep and emotional and financial strain to erode your once positive and bright outlook day to day. Happiness levels appear to bottom out in mid life, with potentially significant and adverse consequences for your mental and physical health. The opportunity for you is to see this mid point of your life as a turning point – a good time to re-evaluate, recalibrate and orient yourself towards what you really want in life. An opportunity for you to reboot your mindset and body to achieve your lifelong goals.

If you're 40-something and battling weight gain or trying to lower chronically elevated blood pressure or blood sugar levels, this book is for you. If you're 40-something and struggling with low energy, frustrated by weight-loss plateaus or the idea of following 'food rules' for the rest of your life, this book is for you.

If you're a personal trainer who works with clients in their mid-30s, 40s and 50s to help them lose weight and improve their energy levels, this book is for you. If you're a practitioner helping people in mid life to improve their health in their mid-30s, 40s and 50s, this book is for you.

What Does PEAK40 Mean?

PEAK40 is about achieving your best health and conquering your performance goals in mid life. The challenge is that lack of sleep, high stress, a demanding schedule and lack of time seem to keep you stuck in neutral (or sometimes what feels like reverse!). Weight gain, fatigue, joint pain and the like, seem to creep up on you and, before you know it, you're battling just to live pain free. This downward spiral can also wreak havoc on your mood and mindset. But it's not just about weight loss, better energy levels and achieving performance milestones (although you will get all that), it's about re-discovering the best version of YOU!

PEAK40 is about simple, evidence-based and time-efficient strategies to help you re-ignite your energy and your passion. Small changes, done consistently over time, yield incredible results. These improve your blood sugar levels, lower high blood pressure, help to avoid heart disease and lose weight to ensure you feel your best today, but also lay the foundations for better health and longevity down the road. Mid life lets you know very quickly that you're no longer indestructible; chronic conditions, like diabetes, hypertension, heart disease or low mood, also infiltrate with no remorse. The years add up and the inflammatory noise in your body begins to drown out the key signals for health and well-being. And it's not just your physical health; your mental health also gets heavily tested. No matter what your level of professional or financial success, science tells us people are always looking up at 'what's next', rather than appreciating how far they've come. PEAK40 isn't just about a physical transformation, but a mindset shift, as well. Re-assess your values, reset expectations and orient yourself towards your lifelong goals. The right mindset ignites the journey – I'll guide you through the process.

The PEAK40 Plan

To get back on track, you first need to shape your path. Do it the right way and you will develop the habits that will set you up for long-term success. It likely took you many months, if not many years, to get to where you are at, so give yourself 6–12 months to reach your PEAK health and performance.

Your plan to PEAK40 health:
Step 1: Master Your Morning
Step 2: Own Your Night
Step 3: Set Your Protein
Step 4: Turn the Dials on Carbs and Fats

Your plan to PEAK40 performance:
Step 1: Restore Your Aerobic Fitness
Step 2: Rebuild Your Muscular Strength *through time-efficient training plans*
Step 3: Upgrade Your Sleep
Step 4: Learn the Right Mindset Skills and Kick-Start Your Path to Happiness – *Mindset is the Keystone to Success*

What You'll Find in This Book

In Section One: *The Downward Spiral*, you'll learn how mindset shifts in mid life and how happiness levels can naturally ebb. You'll see the ripple effects this has on other areas of your life – your activity levels, your food choices and your attitude – and how this also erodes your positive outlook, preventing you from disengaging from negative thoughts and making you more prone to more emotional outbursts. You'll learn how gradual (or not so gradual) accumulation of weight gain over the years can steamroll in mid life into more significant concerns, increasing your risk of high blood pressure, heart disease, metabolic conditions like Type 2 diabetes and certain cancers. Weight gain and obesity don't just have wide-ranging adverse physical effects, but mental effects as well.[1] When your blood glucose levels are chronically elevated, you are at much greater risk of low mood and depression, stoking the fires of chronic inflammation that wreak havoc on health and mental well-being. Inflammation is a protective mechanism to help the body repair. However, poor health leads to an over-active chronic inflammatory response that exacerbates the problem (rather than solving it).

In Section Two: *Nutrition: Shape the Path*, you'll learn how changing your behaviour around nutrition is far more powerful than following a specific dietary plan. You'll navigate all the noise around intermittent fasting, time-restricted eating (TRE) and whether skipping breakfast is better than eating it regularly. You'll learn about the new science to do with late-night eating, how more than 40 per cent of all the calories we consume today come after 6pm and simple tips to curb late-night eating. From there, you'll learn why protein intake really is so crucial to mid-life health and performance, before shifting the focus to how you can effectively manage the rest of your diet – carbohydrates and fats. Building habits is fundamental to reversing poor health or weight gain in mid life. It also sets you up for success in the long-term because you no longer have to make 'food decisions' at every turn; you just do what you do.

In Section Three: *Rebuild and Recover*, you'll learn how to be more efficient with your exercise in mid life. For some, physical activity in mid life grinds to a halt, due to chronic pain and discomfort. For others, lack of time suffocates your attempt to get active. Before you know it, your days are largely sedentary and it starts to show through more aches and pains, deep fatigue, poor sleep, lower libido and mood, just to name a few. It doesn't have to be that way, though. You were born to walk, run, squat, sprint and laugh along the way. Movement is supposed to be fun, not another item on your to-do list. I'll show you how to achieve maximum benefit with the minimum-effective dose and share with you why sleep and recovery strategies, like cold plunges and hot tubs, can catapult you over fitness and weight-loss plateaus.

In Section Four: *Unlock Your Potential*, you'll learn how the biggest hurdle to achieving your goals is the six inches between your ears. The challenges of mid life can create a more negative, anxious and pessimistic mindset. You've misplaced the youthful awe and adventure that kept you effervescent. Taking the time to reflect – about who you are, what your values are and whether your daily actions are in alignment with those targets – is a fundamental part of the process. Knowing yourself becomes a crucial piece of the behaviour-change puzzle. After all, if you can attach a value to why you're making a behaviour change, it's far more likely to stick. Sadly though, in the fast lane of mid life, few people make the time to do it. This is where the mindset skills, like improving your ability to maintain attention, positive self-talk and optimism, are crucial because they allow you the space to reflect, reset and orient yourself in the right direction. Ultimately, if you want to take your nutrition and exercise game to the next level and achieve PEAK40 health and performance, a new mindset will ignite the process.

Peak Strategies for Long-Term Success

The issues facing us today, like climate change and chronic health conditions, such as the obesity epidemic, are increasingly complex and solving such complex problems requires a broader, more holistic view compared to traditional thinking.

The ability to combine solutions from diverse fields – like sleep, medicine, nutrition, training, recovery and mindset – is critical for generating innovative, long-term solutions to 'wicked' problems.[2]

Professor Sidney Dekker, PhD, an expert in complexity and systems thinking, says, 'You cannot reduce a complex system to one of its parts, because if you do, you will tragically and dramatically oversimplify things.' The outcome of a system is never produced by one single part; rather, the outcome is produced via the interactions of all the parts. There is no magic bullet, secret recipe or switch to flip in order to achieve your goals in mid life. There is only effort, consistency and following an evidence-based plan. The path to the finish line is not linear, but if you commit to the process (and not the outcome) and to developing the right habits (not fast-tracking), you'll reach PEAK40 health and performance.

Kind vs. Wicked Learning

Reclaiming your health, body and performance in mid life is not a 'kind' process. A kind learning environment is one in which the outcome is immediate. It provides you with the instant feedback you need to find the correct solution. Golf may not seem like a 'kind' learning environment, but it is. After you hit a shot, the result is right there in front of you. If you understand the golf swing, you can correct the error instantly. In 'kind' learning environments, you can choose a strategy first, then evaluate. It's a very linear process; computers excel in 'kind' environments with less uncertainty and ambiguity.

'Wicked' learning environments have far greater complexity, greater ambiguity and greater uncertainty. 'Wicked' environments require you to evaluate (extensively) first, then choose a strategy. Most challenging of all, the feedback is *not* immediate. You often don't realize you're learning or making progress until days, weeks or months down the road. Managing chronic diseases like hypertension, diabetes and heart disease are all examples of 'wicked' environments. Weight loss is another great example; results are not immediate and the path is not clear. In mid life, the problems you're attempting to solve are 'wicked' – they're complex, they're uncertain and they're ambiguous. It will take time and you may not know, feel or realize you're on the right path until much further down the road. This is known as deep learning.

The Rider and the Elephant

In their terrific book *Switch*, Chip and Dan Heath use the metaphor of the Rider and the Elephant to describe how people make decisions.[3] The Rider is the analytical, data-driven, thinking part of your brain located in the cortex; the Elephant is the emotional brain (the limbic system). Sitting atop the Elephant, the Rider can certainly steer the animal in a desired direction, but only for a certain period of time. The reality is that you can't escape emotion. Dr Tara Swart, MD, PhD, is quick to point out that all your thoughts travel through your limbic system, where they're bathed in emotion, before they reach your cortex for rational analysis. You cannot separate the two. The enormous power and size of the Elephant means that, at any given moment, if it really wants to, it can seize control and the Rider is at its mercy. Expert psychologist Dr John Sullivan, PsyD, with decades of experience working in elite sport, emphasizes to his clients, 'Emotions run the show in sport and in life.' If you want to change behaviours, you need to control the Elephant. How can you do it? Chip and Dan Heath call it 'shaping the path'.

Creating the right environment shapes the path for the Elephant. What looks like a people problem is often a situation problem. You need to nudge the Elephant in the right direction. To motivate the Elephant and lead it down the desired path, you need to 'see' and 'feel' the change you're looking for. It's not enough to know why you should be doing it. You know smoking is bad. You know exercising more will help you lose weight. You know eating less junk food or drinking less alcohol will improve your health. So why do you still do it? You're relying too heavily on the Rider, on your analytical brain and sheer willpower to achieve the desired result. But willpower is a finite resource. You only have so much discipline, and when you run out (and you will run out, especially in mid life), you'll make poor decisions. Why? Because you're human. Elite athletes and Olympians don't jump out of bed at 5.30am because they're always inspired, motivated or even disciplined. If they had to rely on the sparks of inspiration or motivation or the match light of discipline, they would never achieve world-class success. So how do they do it? They repeat behaviours so consistently that the habits become embedded in their DNA. They don't even ask themselves 'if' they should get out of bed, it's automatic; they just do it. I'll show you how to start to shape your path.

Signal vs. Noise

The final theme you'll hear repeated throughout this book is signal versus noise. Signal versus noise is a measure used in science and engineering that compares the level of a desired signal to the level of background noise. For example, try talking to your partner while your child is screaming in the background; the signal (intended message) cannot be communicated effectively because the background noise (child screaming) is too loud. What does this have to do with your health and performance in mid life? Everything. If you're overweight, lacking sleep or struggling with high blood sugar levels, it creates a background level of chronic inflammatory noise. When poor health drives up the inflammatory noise, the body struggles to receive the appropriate signal. This is a problem because usually inflammation is a signal for your body to adapt and grow stronger to fight off a cold or flu, for example, or to grow following exercise. Sometimes, the best way to get your message across isn't to shout louder, it's to stop the screaming in the background. Reducing processed food intake, losing weight and improving glucose control will all help to reduce the inflammatory noise that is scrambling your mental and physical health in mid life.

A Little about Me

I'm a performance nutritionist, naturopathic doctor, former strength and conditioning coach, husband and father of three beautiful little girls, all under the age of seven. (So, I'm right there with you in the hurricane of mid life!)

In my first book, *Peak: The New Science of Athletic Performance That Is Revolutionizing Sports*, I outlined the key fundamentals of elite athletes and high performers *actually* working on the front lines (and not just in an Instagram feed). Why? The gap between what the best of the best athletes and coaches do and what you see 'influencers' doing online is enormous. Athletes will be training with a heavy emphasis on the fundamentals (not the fads), on consistency (not extreme effort) and on the value of patience (not rapid transformation). No wonder so many clients struggle with achieving their goals.

I haven't written *Peak 40* for you to transform your life into some artificial, unrealistic Instagram-able ideal, but as a practical guide to navigating mid life so you can thrive in it (and not just survive).

The Downward Spiral

CHAPTER 1

The Mid-Life Happiness Curve

'Happiness is a direction, not a place.'

— SYDNEY J. HARRIS, journalist and author

What does happiness have to do with achieving your best health and performance in mid life? Why does it matter? Tackling complex problems, like weight gain or a chronic health condition, requires consistency and patience. They take time to resolve. Why? They require you to change behaviours in your life, such as what you eat, how much (and how intensely) you move, how much you sleep, and so on. These behaviours are much more deeply rooted than you may think, which is why you can't always change them overnight. Behaviour change is difficult. To make the road a little smoother and give you the greatest odds of staying on track in the long run, you need the right mindset. You need the right attitude to empower your effort; you need the right thoughts to trigger the desired actions. Happiness helps ignite the process. In fact, performance psychologists in elite sport have turned the old adage of 'achieve success and happiness will follow' on its head, with a new model of aiming for happiness first, in order to propel behaviour change and *then* success.

The Mid-Life U-Shaped Happiness Curve

Dr David Blanchflower, Professor of Economics at Dartmouth University, and his team examined the well-being data in 132 countries with respect to 15 measures of unhappiness – fatigue, sadness, strain, tension, anxiety, depression, sleeplessness, etc – and uncovered a U-shaped 'happiness curve'.[1] Happiness levels appear to start out very high in childhood and adolescence (not surprising), but after the age of 18, Blanchflower found happiness levels begin to decrease steadily until into mid life. In fact, happiness levels appear to reach their lowest point between the ages of 41 to 47 years old in developed countries. (That seems like an awfully big chunk of mid life!) Blanchflower found happiness levels steadily increase in your late 40s and continue to do so well into your 70s (thus the 'U-shaped' curve). Remarkably, the relationship held true even when researchers controlled for gender, education, marital status and social class.

You may be wondering how this evidence could hold up across so many different countries and continents. In the 95 developing and 37 advanced countries his team analyzed, the U-shaped happiness curve was consistently found in North and South America, Europe, Asia, Australasia and Africa. It even held true in countries where people live longer and in countries where people do not. It seems odd that in mid life, when most individuals have some levels of financial security, happiness levels would be so low. Doesn't money bring more happiness? Not exactly. Interestingly, the U-shape relationship remained constant in countries with both high and low median wages – your financial position isn't much of a factor when it comes to happiness.

While it's nice to hear things will get better as you age, you probably don't want to spend your 40s in the doldrums waiting for the fog to lift naturally in your late 40s. Does this really mean you're destined for a decade of unhappiness? The good news is that happiness is a trainable skill, and the more skilled you become, the greater the likelihood it will propel you to higher performance in all aspects of your life.

Why Does Happiness Dip in Mid Life?

Why might happiness drop in mid life? Blanchflower and his team offer a few possible explanations. The first is our inherent drive for 'success'. Young and ambitious in your 20s and early 30s, you steamroll ahead motivated to achieve your career goals. No doubt this brings a sense of satisfaction and pride, but, ironically, the sensation doesn't last very long. Researchers call this hedonic adaptation.[2] Once you achieve your goal, the celebration is short-lived and your successes unconsciously move the goalposts forward. No matter what your level of success, you're always looking up the ladder of achievement at what needs to be accomplished next (and you forget to look back in the rear-view mirror often enough to enjoy how far you've come). Why is this problematic? Because the 'happiness', like the celebration from achievement, is short-lived. In fact, some people may even feel guilt or shame because they don't feel happy as a result of their career and financial success; a sense of ungratefulness, which further exacerbates mid-life dissatisfaction.

The next possible explanation for low mid-life happiness comes down to expectations. When you're young, the world is your oyster. You have the benefit of time and can look forward to achieving your ambitions. But life doesn't always play out as you imagine it to. You may not achieve all your career goals. You may find the physical and emotional toll of caring for young children and ageing parents far more taxing than you ever imagined. It can take some time to come to terms with your new outlook on life. It's not just the constant pursuit of achievement or expectations that can alter your world view, comparisons to friends or colleagues may also begin to sting as you age. Comparison drives competition and, ironically, this appears to hinder your sense of satisfaction with your efforts. In your 40s, because you feel you have less ability to change the situation, it can erode your confidence and impact on your identity. There will always be someone fitter, wealthier or higher up the career ladder than you (and thanks to social media, you've probably heard of them!). This leads to a series of negative feedback loops in the brain, enhancing negative self-talk and thoughts, which can dampen your mood and zest for life.

Is Happiness Genetic?

You probably know a magnetic person – a colleague, coach or famous athlete or entertainer – whose mere presence energizes the whole group. Are these people just the lucky ones? Is it possible to be a genetically happy person? It's a great question; one scientists have explored. Genetics does appear to play a large role in your baseline happiness levels. A landmark research project called the Minnesota Twin Family Study, conducted from 1979 to 1999, followed identical and fraternal twins who were separated from their biological parents not long after birth and raised in different homes.[3] The study is unique because it provides a glimpse into how genes versus environment impact key areas of personality (including baseline happiness). When researchers assessed happiness, they found the happiness levels of identical twins were almost always exactly the same, despite the fact they were separated at birth. Results were not the same for fraternal twins, who do not share exactly the same DNA; they were found to have significantly different baseline happiness levels. To sum up, there is indeed a genetic 'baseline' level of happiness.

But genetics is only one part of the happiness equation. What else contributes? You might presume that the obvious external factors in your life, such as income, money, job status, social status, house, etc, were high on the list. Not quite. Material possessions aren't nearly as strong a factor as you might think. A comparison of the richest people in America by *Forbes* magazine found the top 1 per cent of the country are only marginally happier than average. (Incredibly, about one third of the top 1 per cent were actually less happy than average.) Money does matter to a certain point, though. External circumstances account for approximately one third of your happiness. What's the last third of happiness? Your mindset.

Emotions Run the Show

You might think that you make decisions based on logic, but the best performance psychologists in the world are quick to point out this isn't the case. Dr Peter Jensen, PhD, mental performance coach to countless Olympians says, '90 per cent of the decisions you make are based on emotion.'[4] What effect is your mindset having on your physical health? What effect is your mindset having on sustaining your diet and exercise choices? What effect is your mindset having on your sleep, nutrition, movement, recovery and mental health? The trickle-down effects on your ability to thrive at work, at home and in life are highly significant. Your mindset can propel you to PEAK40 health and performance, or it can sabotage your success and leave you feeling stuck.

Lead Your Elephant down the Right Path

Performance psychologists also call attention to the fact that there are very few things you can *actually* control. What can you control? It's a very short list: attitude, actions, effort and thoughts. That's all. Attitude, actions and effort are the 'easiest' to wrestle control over; the Rider can steer these in the right direction through sheer willpower alone. Controlling your thoughts, however, is more challenging (the domain of the Elephant). Willpower and effort alone are not enough to overpower the Elephant and change its course. The Elephant is too powerful. How can you steer the Elephant to where you want it to go? You must create the right environment, the right path for the Elephant to follow. This is where most people go wrong, they rely on brute force and relentless effort. It's time to learn a better way.

The right mindset empowers you to take action and make yourself accountable for what you eat, how much (or little) you move and your lifestyle choices, like sleep, that impact not only how you look, feel and perform every day, but ultimately your happiness level. The great challenge in mid life, when trying to control your emotions (and the thoughts that emerge as a result), are the major roadblocks, like always being 'busy', chronic high stress, lack of sleep and constant fatigue. All of these factors are strongly associated with lower mid-life happiness and they all compromise your mental health.

Consider for a moment the importance of sleep for mental and physical health. Lack of sleep is associated with a greater risk of depressed mood and chronic conditions, like hypertension and pre-diabetes, not to mention the expected fatigue and daytime sleepiness.[5] Insufficient sleep has also been shown to impair your ability to disengage from negative thoughts.[6] This can quickly unravel into poor food and lifestyle choices, like opting out of your exercise regime, all of which then adversely influence your mental health.[7] The downward spiral of negative self-talk can make changing your habits feel like climbing Mount Everest – the summit is so far away, why even bother trying?

If you take a holistic view of low mood and depression, you realize a myriad of factors contribute to low mood – lack of sleep, high stress, poor glucose control, weight gain, chronic inflammation and lack of aerobic fitness. For example, higher blood glucose levels in mid life can impact your mental health as much as your physical health. A study in *Diabetes Care* of over 4,000 people showed depressive symptoms were highly associated with higher fasting insulin levels – a biomarker of poor diet and metabolic health.[8] (In fact, the authors specifically noted that antidepressant medications did not alter this association). In Scandinavia, researchers found a clear association between elevated HbA1c – a three-month average of blood sugar levels – with increased risk of depression.[9] These results highlight that poor diet, and the subsequent elevation in your blood sugar levels, creates a milieu where low mood and depression can take root. If your blood sugar levels are consistently high or if you're overweight or unfit, it can also quickly lead to a chronic state of low-grade inflammation. The prestigious *New England Journal of Medicine* recently published a review highlighting the strong connection between chronic inflammation and the development of depression, high blood pressure, pre-diabetes and most common chronic diseases.[10] If you are overweight or obese (defined as a body mass index [BMI] of 30kg/m^2 or more) in mid life, you likely have some kind of chronic low-grade inflammation adversely impacting your mental state. When the internal inflammatory fires burn too intensely, they begin to erode both your physical and mental health. Your state of subpar physical health and fitness, as well as the high demands and hectic pace of mid life, can create a current that is pulling you downstream towards a pessimistic mindset and lower levels of happiness. Reversing this current is a key step to reclaiming PEAK40 health and performance.

CHAPTER 2

Super Bowl or Heart Attack?

'To achieve success, whatever the job we have, we must pay a price.'
— VINCE LOMBARDI, American football coach

Winning a Super Bowl is a once in a lifetime opportunity. Athletes and coaches work tirelessly throughout their careers for the mere opportunity to reach the pinnacle of their sport. In the 1980s, Dan Reeves was the head coach of the NFL's Denver Broncos, one of the league's premier teams, playing in three Super Bowls that decade. Unfortunately for coach Reeves and the Broncos, they lost all three. However, the heartache and disappointment of 'almost' achieving a championship trophy didn't deter Reeves from pursuing the ultimate prize.

In the early 1990s, Reeves left the Broncos to take on the challenge of bringing a winning culture to the moribund Atlanta Falcons franchise. The Falcons had suffered through eight losing seasons in the 80s and were consistently one of the worst teams in American football. Reeves brought his tireless work ethic and tenacity to Atlanta, working late nights and early mornings over the next few years, before turning the Falcons around into a respected, competitive team. By 1998, Reeves had built the Falcons into a championship contender; they were on the verge of making a serious run for the Super Bowl. Then, suddenly, it all changed. Not for the Falcons, but for coach Reeves. In late December, Reeves felt an intense burning sensation in his throat. Begrudgingly, he called his doctor and made an appointment for the next day.

When Reeves met with his cardiologist, the doctor informed Reeves he was in serious trouble and that his heart needed urgent surgery. A fierce competitor on the precipice of achieving a life-long goal, Reeves did the unthinkable; he dismissed the warning. Coach Reeves wanted to put off treatment until the season was complete so he could finish the job in hand with the Falcons. The cardiologist responded sharply, telling him bluntly that his heart could fail at any moment, that he could have a heart attack and die that night. Reeves finally relented; he had quadruple bypass surgery that same day.

Of course, coach Reeve's poor cardiovascular health didn't happen overnight. In his mid 40s, he had multiple angioplasties – a medical procedure used to widen narrow or obstructed arteries – commonly used to treat atherosclerosis. Like most chronic conditions, what you eat, how much (or little) you move and lifestyle factors, like sleep, play fundamental roles in the years and decades leading up to a major event like a heart attack or stroke. Striving for PEAK40 health and performance isn't just about looking good physically, it's about protecting yourself from the chronic conditions that can quickly derail your mental and physical health.

Atherosclerosis: The Silent Killer

Cardiovascular disease (CVD) is an umbrella term used to describe a wide range of disorders affecting your heart and blood vessels, such as atherosclerosis, hypertension, stroke and peripheral artery and vein diseases.[1] Globally, CVD is the number one cause of mortality, accounting for over 30 per cent of all disease-related deaths. The good news is that rates of heart attack and stroke don't reach their highest point until your mid 50s, but what you do (or don't do) in your 40s will play a key role in managing your risk. To achieve PEAK40 health, keeping your heart and vessels strong is non-negotiable.

What causes heart attacks and strokes? There is no one single cause. However, a hallmark indication of disease progression is atherosclerosis, the narrowing of your arteries. It's one of the most fundamental processes in the development of heart disease. If you can fight off atherosclerosis, you'll protect your heart for years to come. But atherosclerosis is a 'silent killer', meaning early warning signs are so subtle they often go unnoticed. If you have mildly elevated blood pressure readings, this may be your first clue to take action.

The narrowing of your arteries also increases your blood pressure. Chronically elevated blood pressure is a big problem because it increases the risk of damaging the delicate innermost lining of your arterial walls called the endothelium and, in turn, this kicks off a chronic inflammatory process, which leads to further narrowing and stiffening of your arteries, putting you at major risk of heart attack or stroke.[2]

Dyslipidaemia – abnormal amounts of lipids in the blood (high LDL-cholesterol [LDL-c], high triglycerides and/or low HDL-cholesterol [HDL-c]) – is also linked to increased risk of heart disease, but it is just one of the messengers. Weight gain and chronically elevated blood glucose levels are the primary root causes – the loudest 'signals' – promoting chronic inflammation, platelet adhesion (making your red blood cells stickier) and sending those biomarkers out of balance. The combination of plaque formation (laid down to repair damaged arteries), oxidative stress (an imbalance of free radicals and antioxidants caused by poor diet and lifestyle) and inflammation is the triple threat that dramatically increases your risk of heart attack and stroke.

Can You Outrun a Bad Diet?

Coach Dan Reeves, like most NFL coaches, was a former pro football player. In the mid 1960s and early 70s, Reeves played eight seasons with the legendary Dallas Cowboys, culminating in a Super Bowl win over the Miami Dolphins in 1971. Playing professional football requires impressive speed, strength and size. Reeves was a running back, a skill-position typically characterized by speed and a lower body-fat percentage. In stark contrast, the burly offensive and defensive linemen require more brute strength and power to survive the pounding in the trenches at the line of scrimmage on every play. To achieve their impressive power and strength, offensive and defensive linemen must put on a significant amount of body weight – both muscle and fat – to deliver powerful blocks and ferocious hits on opposing players.

The problem for your heart is that gaining a lot of weight is a serious issue. When your body mass index (BMI) exceeds 30kg/m^2 – the medical definition of obesity – this is a strong *independent* predictor of a heart attack or stroke.[3]

A study of over 500 professional American football players found offensive and defensive linemen had a mean BMI of 31.4, placing them in the 'obese' category (significantly higher than the skill positions, like Reeves and wide receivers).[4] Professional NFL football players are elite athletes with impressive levels of fitness and muscle mass, both well-recognized traits that are highly beneficial for your vascular and heart health. Despite their size, NFL linemen have markedly good metabolic health biomarkers on blood tests. But what happens when they retire and stop exercising so regularly (and vigorously)? It's very similar to what happens to the rest of us in mid life when we stop exercising because the demands of the day have filled up all the available hours (and then some!). We get fat! Let's take a closer look.

In the 1990s, the first analysis of heart disease mortality in former NFL players was conducted by the National Institute for Occupational Safety and Health.[5] Over 6,800 players were tested and researchers found 'all-cause mortality' (i.e. death by any cause) was 46 per cent lower among former pro football players compared to the general population. This makes sense, athletes have higher fitness levels and more muscle mass compared to the average person, a great recipe for longevity. Unfortunately, upon closer inspection, something more troubling was uncovered. When scientists looked specifically at *former* offensive and defensive linemen, cardiovascular disease mortality shot up by a whopping 52 per cent. If you were a lineman with a BMI of 30 or more during your years of active play, you had almost *double the risk* of cardiovascular disease mortality compared with other former players (primarily attributable to atherosclerosis and high blood pressure). A follow-up study in 2012 yielded similar results.[6]

It's Not Just about Weight

Weight gain is tightly linked to high blood pressure, which of course plays a strong role in atherosclerosis and arterial damage. It's also connected to chronically high blood glucose levels, another strong risk factor for cardiovascular disease. One of the first studies to identify this relationship was a 22-year observational study that found when fasting blood glucose exceeded 85mg/dl (4.7mmol/L), it was associated with a 40 per cent increased risk of cardiovascular disease (after correcting for all variables that skew the association).[7] Similarly, the Whitehall study of over 19,000 male civil servants in London (aged 40–69 when first examined in the late 1960s) was set up at the height of the vascular disease epidemic in the UK to assess for key risk factors in an attempt to predict heart disease mortality. What did they uncover? Researchers found an increased risk of cardiovascular disease with the highest fasting glucose values, which itself increased in a step-wise fashion as fasting blood glucose worsened.[8] The higher your fasting levels, the worse your health was likely to be. Perhaps most worrying was that the association was strongest in men aged 40–49. These findings also hold strong after correcting for age, cholesterol, systolic blood pressure, obesity and smoking.[9]

What about Wine and Beer?

What about the effects of alcohol on heart health? Let's review. Red wine is a top-10 polyphenol-rich food providing an impressive 126mg per serving.[10] (Note – pinot noir and cabernet sauvignon are among the highest polyphenol red wines.) The polyphenols found in a glass of wine help to reduce the harmful *oxidized* LDL-c and increase nitric oxide, promoting vasodilation (the widening of blood vessels) and improving your arterial health. Furthermore, red wine also increases protective HDL-c levels, inhibits the aggregation of platelets (reducing the 'stickiness' of your RBCs), promotes the breakdown of fibrous clots and reduces inflammation, all of which help fight off the progression of atherosclerosis.[11]

For middle-aged women, wine consumption appears to be protective against heart disease. A recent study of 2,900 culturally diverse, healthy women found moderate wine consumption (equal to one glass of wine per day) lowered inflammatory CRP and fibrinogen (clotting) levels compared to women who drank little wine or abstained completely.[12] These are all major wins for *modest* amounts of red wine in your diet. But while one glass of wine may support good health, if you've finished the entire bottle (imbibed nightly!), things start to unravel quickly. Excess wine consumption will compromise blood sugar control, quality of sleep and ultimately increase your heart disease risk.

What about beer? Beer gets a bad rap when it comes to 'healthy' alcohol options. Let's be honest, the 'beer belly' isn't exactly the best marketing campaign. Don't let that fool you, though; beer is another very good source of polyphenols. You might be shocked to learn that low to moderate intakes of beer (one or two 330ml/11.6oz bottles per day) are also shown to be protective against heart disease and its effects are actually comparable to red wine.[13] In 1999, approximately 7,000 British men were recruited and tracked over 17 years to determine how alcohol consumption impacts mortality. How did the beer drinkers fare? Regular beer consumption was associated with lower total mortality (pass the IPA!).[14] But caution, this isn't a carte blanche to knock back all the lagers and stouts you can find – moderate consumption of one to two bottles, three to four times per week, is the key.

Don't forget about non-alcoholic beer – it rehydrates your body faster than water. At the 2018 Winter

Olympics in South Korea, the German national team doctors used non-alcoholic beer to help athletes rehydrate after training and events.[15] Johannes Scherr, team doctor for the German Olympic ski team, found in his earlier research at the Technical University of Munich that athletes who drank non-alcoholic beer had fewer upper respiratory infections compared to a placebo because the beer provides key micronutrients for immunity. It also contains the health-promoting polyphenols, shown to lower pro-inflammatory homocysteine, IL-6 and TNF-B levels.[16] The Krombacher brewery delivered 3,500 litres of non-alcoholic beer to the German team in the athletes' village in Pyeongchang. That's a serious rehydration strategy!

Finally, weight gain impacts high blood pressure via an altogether different mechanism. A common root cause that gets much less attention is the effect of chronically high insulin on blood pressure, via its impact on the hormone aldosterone. Aldosterone is a hormone secreted by the adrenal glands that sit atop your kidneys, whose role is to regulate electrolyte and water levels in your body. When aldosterone levels are high, it signals your kidneys to retain more sodium and thus more water. This in turn increases your blood volume and ultimately your blood pressure. When you're in good health, your body naturally lowers aldosterone levels to clear the excess salt via the kidneys. If your insulin levels are chronically high due to high blood sugar levels or weight gain, aldosterone levels stay chronically high leading to high blood pressure. As the pressure rises inside your vessels, your arterial walls begin to thicken, further exacerbating the high blood pressure cycle. Dr Ben Bikman, PhD, insulin scientist, sums things up nicely stating, 'insulin resistance' – chronically elevated insulin levels – 'is a key feature in hypertension and CVD risk for most people.'[17]

In Summary

In mid life, poor food choices, lack of sleep and weight gain can also conspire against you to start to sabotage your vascular health. The two major culprits contributing to this downward spiral are excess energy (calorie) intake and physical inactivity. Both factors are key drivers of weight gain and obesity. The good news is that there is a large body of evidence to suggest that good nutrition may be the most preventative factor for CVD events, possibly even powerful enough to reverse heart disease.[18] You can start to bulletproof your heart health with a strategic combination of nutrition, exercise and weight loss.

How did coach Reeves' Falcons do in 1998 in their quest for a Super Bowl win after he suffered his quadruple bypass? Atlanta finished strong winning the division and upsetting the heavily favoured Minnesota Vikings in the conference final to make it to the Super Bowl. Incredibly, coach Reeves recovered in time, with medical team support and a series of diet and exercise strategies, to coach his team from the sidelines in the Super Bowl. While the Falcons didn't win the big game, the lessons Reeves learned have helped keep him healthy today at the age of 76. You don't have to choose between *your* 'Super Bowl' and your health. There is a better way.

CHAPTER 3

The Blood-Sugar Rollercoaster

'What looks like a people problem is often a situation problem.'
— DAN HEATH, author and researcher

It's 2018. Tyronn Lue, the 41-year-old head coach of the National Basketball Association's Cleveland Cavaliers, is experiencing significant chest pain and coughing up blood. Coming out of half time, his symptoms worsen and he's unable to coach the rest of the game. Lue has guided the Cavaliers to three straight NBA finals, winning in historic fashion in 2016 with the help of LeBron James – the best basketball player in the world – where the team rallied from a three-games-to-one deficit (a first!), against the heavily favoured Golden State Warriors. They lost to the Warriors in 2017 and so the goal in 2018 was to return to the finals and win another championship. But Lue was also experiencing significant anxiety, persistent fatigue and rarely getting a full night's sleep, due to the demands of the job. The battery of tests performed by the team's medical staff confirmed his heart was fine, but that Lue was suffering from burnout. His lack of sleep, high stress levels and poor diet laden with processed convenience foods and soda pop had caught up with him. Reluctantly, Lue took a leave of absence from the team to address his health.

Your environment has the biggest influence on your health. Not just the hectic, high-stress environment of professional coaching, but today's processed food environment that amplifies blood sugar dysregulation, weight gain and inflammation. The normal human physiological response is to crave sugar when stressed. What's abnormal? Having calorie-dense, nutrient-poor foods around you 24/7. Lue is the first to admit his food choices hastened his ill health. Let's explore how today's food environment is impacting your waistline and health.

The Mid-Life Weight Gain

For many, weight gain seems to appear overnight as you hit your 40s. Of course, this is just an illusion. The realization you've gained weight may hit you in one swift blow, but the likelihood is that extra weight around your mid section took years to get there; at least, that's what the science says. Scientists recently crunched the numbers from two large studies in the United States that followed approximately 25,000 men and 90,000 women over multiple decades. Study participants recorded their weight in young adulthood – aged 18 for women and 21 for men – and continued until the age of 55. What did the data reveal? On average, the women gained an additional 28 pounds (12.7kg) over the 37-year timespan, while men put on 21 extra pounds (9.5kg) over 34 years.[1] What's interesting is that both groups gained weight very gradually over time. This makes sense; you start adding a couple of pounds (1kg) a year in your late 20s, it continues throughout your 30s, and all of a sudden you hit 40 and realize you're holding on to 10, 20 or 30 plus extra pounds.

Weighing It Up

Adult weight gain is consistently connected to a higher risk of Type 2 diabetes, heart disease, high blood pressure and several types of cancer.[2] What's surprising in this new line of research is that even gradual weight gain – that extra 20 pounds over the years – also puts you at greater risk of chronic conditions. To put things into perspective, for every 4.5kg/10lb increase in weight gain, there is a 17 per cent reduction in your odds of ageing well. Not the statistics you want to hear in mid life.

Most chronic conditions begin to accelerate in your 40s and worsen with weight gain. By the time Americans reach mid life, 90 per cent will struggle with hypertension and 40 per cent will suffer from metabolic syndrome, a cluster of symptoms including high blood pressure, high blood sugar, excess body fat around the belly and abnormal cholesterol or triglyceride levels.[3]

In short, weight gain in adulthood is not benign. The message is clear; if you don't take action in your 40s, your health will be compromised (in a very serious way). The good news is that weight loss, on its own, is the most powerful 'signal' for improving glucose control and reversing Type 2 diabetes. But weight gain is less to do with 'getting older' and more to do with being set in your ways; your old habits are hard to change. The Elephant doesn't want to listen to the Rider.

You May Think You're Healthy ...

Chronically high blood glucose levels can still sabotage your health, even if you're healthy. A hallmark study followed approximately 2,000 healthy, non-diabetic men aged 40–59 for over two decades and uncovered that men with higher fasting glucose levels had significantly greater mortality rate from heart disease.[4] They concluded that fasting blood glucose values in the upper normal range – not outside the normal range – appears to be an important *independent* predictor of cardiovascular death in non-diabetic, healthy, middle-aged men. This should be an eye-opener for all men over 40. Even if you're not overweight, if your blood glucose levels are in the upper normal range, it's time to take action.

What should you be aiming for when it comes to blood glucose control, health and longevity? If you visit your doctor for an annual physical, they'll assess your fasting glucose levels. If all your numbers come back in the normal range, you'll get the all-clear and likely not hear back from your doctor. While it's great you've passed the first benchmark – achieving glucose levels in the 'normal' range – you can gain further insights from knowing your exact fasting glucose score. A recent study in the journal *Diabetes Care* examining 12.8 million people and the relationship between fasting blood glucose and mortality, found that fasting glucose levels between 80–94mg/dL (4.4–5.2mmol/L) were associated with the lowest mortality, regardless of age and sex (see Table 3.1).[5] It appears that fasting glucose might be a pretty good proxy for health status and longevity.

These findings are even more compelling when you consider that the aforementioned study found glucose levels at 100mg/dL (5.6mmol/L) and above were connected with higher mortality. A fasting glucose score of 100mg/dL (5.6mmol/L) is within the traditional 'normal' range of 72–108mg/dL (4.0–6.0mmol/L) that is still used in many parts of the world. If you know your

Table 3.1. Normal, Pre-Diabetic and Diabetic Ranges for Fasting Glucose

	Normal Range	Pre-Diabetes	Diabetes
Fasting (metric)	Below 5.5 mmol/L	5.5–6.9 mmol/L	7.0mmol/L and above
Fasting (USA)	Below 100mg/dl	100–125 mg/dl	126mg/dl and above

score, rather than if you're simply within the range, it can serve as a red flag to let you know it's time to revisit and upgrade your diet, exercise and lifestyle regime.

Another benefit of aiming for a glucose target, rather than following a specific diet, is that you can choose from any dietary strategy. It doesn't matter what dietary strategy you prefer – low-carb, low-fat, paleo, vegan, keto or anything in between – your glucose score gives you an objective assessment of your diet. Remember, all diets operate under the same set of rules, there is no 'magic' diet. The magic is in building the right habits.

Assess Your Environment

How can you start to fight off blood sugar highs and lows, poor energy and weight gain? Willpower is one option, but remember, it's a finite resource. The Elephant will always be much more powerful. The best strategy, therefore, is to create an environment where it is easy for the Elephant to follow the path.

Nutrition is complex and recommendations can seem quite polarizing, even among expert scientists and doctors. Let's start with what most expert health associations agree on – what *not* to eat. The leading heart, diabetes and cancer associations around the world recommend you avoid:

- high salt
- high refined sugar
- high trans fats

What's the common denominator among these food ingredients? They're found overwhelmingly in ultra-processed foods. Ultimately, these send your blood sugar levels on a rollercoaster ride for the day, shooting up and crashing down. Unfortunately, these peaks and valleys also accelerate weight gain, glucose dysfunction, inflammation and oxidative stress.[6]

Beware of Ultra-processed Foods

There aren't a lot of foods occurring in nature with that combination of high fat and high sugar, but ultra-processed foods contain just the right (wrong) mix of sugar, fat, salt and flavour additives to kick up a dopamine 'reward' signal response in your brain that then makes you crave them.

From Buenos Aires to Boston, and London to Tokyo, ultra-processed foods are becoming the norm worldwide.[7] They now dominate the food landscape, making up the majority of calories we consume.[8] In Brazil, the prevalence of obesity jumped from 7.5 to 17 per cent in a little over a decade (from 2002 to 2013) among adults aged 20–39 years, and from 14.7 to 25.7 per cent among those aged 40–59 years.[9] This led Professor Carlos Monteiro, PhD, from Sao Paulo University in Brazil, and his research team to develop the NOVA diet classification system to put more emphasis on the nature, extent and degree of processing when categorizing foods and beverages (See Table 3.2).

What exactly is an *ultra-processed* food? NOVA defines ultra-processed foods as 'formulations mostly of cheap industrial sources of dietary energy and nutrients plus additives, using a series of processes and containing minimal whole foods'.[10] The NOVA system is divided into four groups: (1) unprocessed or minimally processed foods, (2) processed culinary ingredients, (3) processed foods and (4) ultra-processed foods. In layperson's terms, if it has more than five ingredients, it's probably an ultra-processed food. Rather than the traditional approach to talking calories, macronutrients or even 'animal versus plant', the NOVA system shifts the focus back to the quality of your diet, eating more 'real food'!

Keep It Simple

Like any new system, NOVA has been criticized. There have been accusations that it is too imprecise and incomplete to form

Table 3.2. NOVA Ultra-processed Foods List

Group 1: Unprocessed and Minimally Processed	Leafy and cruciferous vegetables; brown or white rice; legumes, such as beans, lentils and chickpeas; starchy roots and tubers, such as potatoes, sweet potatoes and cassava; meat, poultry, eggs, fish and seafood; milk; fruit or vegetable juices (with no added sugar, sweeteners or flavours); corn, wheat, oats, tree and ground nuts and other oily seeds; plain yogurt; tea, coffee and drinking water.
Group 2: Processed Culinary Ingredients	Vegetable oils crushed from seeds, nuts or fruit (notably olives); butter and lard obtained from milk and pork; sugar and molasses obtained from cane or beet; honey, maple syrup and vegetable oils; sea salt and table salt with added drying agents.
Group 3: Processed Foods	Canned or bottled vegetables and legumes in brine; salted or sugared nuts and seeds; salted, dried, cured or smoked meats and fish; canned fish (with or without added preservatives); fruit in syrup (with or without added antioxidants); freshly made unpackaged breads and cheeses.
Group 4: Ultra-processed Foods	Ready-to-eat products, such as carbonated soft drinks; sweet or savoury packaged snacks; chocolate and confectionery (candies); ice cream; mass-produced packaged breads and buns; margarines and other spreads; biscuits (cookies), pastries, cakes and cake mixes; breakfast cereals, cereal and 'energy' bars; 'energy' drinks; milk drinks, 'fruit' yogurts and 'fruit' drinks; 'cocoa' drinks; 'instant' sauces.

the foundation for making dietary recommendations.[11] That hasn't stopped Brazil's national dietary guidelines from using the NOVA system to combat the rapid rise in weight gain and chronic diseases of lifestyle, and to recommend that ultra-processed foods should be avoided. The beauty of the NOVA system is its simplicity in the complex 'wicked' world of nutrition. What

Belly Fat and a Bad Microbiome

Your gut microbiome – the collection of your gut microbiota community and their genes – plays a critical role in your health. Weight gain, high belly fat and persistently high blood sugar levels disrupt your gut microbiota community, significantly reducing the diversity of your gut microbiome, which acts as an interface between you and the outside world. Scientist Rob Knight, PhD, of the University of California, San Diego, and founder of the American Gut Project, a scientific initiative to map the human gut, refers to the microbiome as a 'microbe organ', due to the profound impact it has on virtually all systems of the body. Incredibly, scientists can now identify Type 2 diabetes patients simply by analyzing the collection of bacteria in their gut. It's little wonder, then, that ultra-processed foods have been shown to disrupt gut-brain signalling and adversely impact your satiety (feeling of fullness), leading to greater food intake when compared to the calories from whole foods. Moreover, a high degree of bacterial diversity is considered to be a potential biomarker of health and longevity.[12] How can you support a healthy gut microbiome in mid life? Maintain a healthy weight, keep good glucose control and eat a wide variety of vegetables, fruit and whole foods.

happens when you reduce your intake of ultra-processed food and eat more 'real' food? Your calorie intake drops (often dramatically). You increase your consumption of vitamins, minerals and key antioxidants. And you increase your intake of fibre.

The problem is ultra-processed foods are highly palatable, making it really easy to over-indulge.[13] It's not simply a lack of willpower that leads to over-consumption, these foods are specifically engineered to have just the right combination of salt, sugar, fat, and the like, to leave you wanting more.[14] They've been masterfully crafted by food scientists to trigger your appetite cues, which for some people, can lead to highly dysfunctional eating behaviours.[15]

Does Ultra-processed Food Cause Weight Gain?

It makes sense that if your diet is made up primarily of ultra-processed foods, you'll inevitably consume more calories and gain more weight. Yet, until recently, there was no scientific smoking gun proving that ultra-processed food causes weight gain. Dr Kevin Hall, PhD, from the National Institute of Diabetes and Digestive and Kidney Diseases (NIDDK) in Bethesda, Maryland, conducted a study with 20 inpatients comparing a minimally processed diet to an ultra-processed diet on health outcomes.[16] How did the 'real food' stack up against all the packaged stuff that lines the middle aisles of grocery stores? Hall and his team recruited 10 men and 10 women who spent four weeks in a metabolic ward at the NIH Metabolic Clinical Research Unit (MCRU). The average age and body mass index (BMI) of participants was 31 and 27kg/m2, respectively. The two groups were randomly assigned to consume either an ultra-processed or minimally processed diet for 14 days before immediately swapping over to the alternative diet. The study participants ate three daily meals and were allowed to eat as much or as little as desired (within an hour). The meals were specifically designed to be matched for total calories, macronutrients, fibre, sugars and sodium, but varied considerably in the percentage of calories derived from ultra-processed versus unprocessed foods.

What happened after 28 days in a metabolic ward? The study participants gained around 0.9kg/2lb on the processed food diet, while those on the unprocessed diet lost about 0.97kg/2.13lb. When participants were eating the ultra-processed diet, they consumed approximately 500 calories more per day and ate at a much faster pace than those on the unprocessed diet. It may seem intuitive, but this study by Hall and his team was the first to demonstrate causality; ultra-processed foods *cause* people to eat too many calories and gain weight. It's not surprising, therefore, that in a food environment where over half of all the food we buy is ultra-processed, we're struggling as a society to maintain a healthy weight.

Fat Plus Sugar Is a Wicked Combination

Hall's colleague, Dr Emma Stinson, PhD, also uncovered that the combination of high fat with high sugar in processed foods *independently predicted* overeating and weight gain.[17] If the food environment in your home, office or even car is laden with ultra-processed options, you'll struggle to succeed. The Elephant will not be able to resist its hardwired evolutionary instinct to seek out calorie-dense sugar and fat when stressed or lacking sleep. (In short, every day of your life in your 40s!)

You might think this is just a North and South American problem; far from it. Travel across the pond to France and a recent study of over 100,000 people found ultra-processed food consumption was strongly associated with an increased risk of

Food Environment Starts at Home

When it comes to losing weight and fighting off Type 2 diabetes in mid life, your partner or spouse may play the most influential role. A recent study in Type 2 diabetics revealed 'spousal concordance' was the strongest factor predicting levels of physical activity and successful dietary changes.[18] The message appears to be clear: be careful who you marry, you'll likely develop similar behaviours. They also found a link between the body weight of one spouse and the risk of diagnosis of Type 2 diabetes in their partner. In contrast, when one spouse loses weight on a weight management programme, the other spouse is also likely to shed weight. All the more reason to achieve PEAK40 health together!

Type 2 diabetes.[19] Perhaps even more troubling, these findings were *independent* of body weight and nutritional quality of the diet (two factors that typically affect Type 2 diabetes risk). Even when participants avoided weight gain from the initial visit to follow-ups, they were still at increased risk of developing diabetes if their ultra-processed consumption was high. Considering blood sugar control typically worsens as you age, it's another red flag to keep your convenience food intake to a minimum if you want to achieve PEAK40 health.

Ultra-processed food consumption is strongly linked to increased risks of cancer, cardiovascular diseases, depression, metabolic disorder, mortality and Type 2 diabetes. All the bad stuff that can take root in mid life. Longer working hours, less sleep and more stress trigger the brain to crave sugar, fat and salt, and our modern ultra-processed food environment has an endless supply. It's not a lack of willpower that leads to weight gain or poor glucose control – accomplished psychologist and behaviour change experts Chip and Dan Heath say, 'What looks like a person problem is actually a situation problem.' When it comes to weight gain and chronic health conditions, it's an ultra-processed food environment problem. However, it's not enough to 'know' something is bad for you. You need to shape the path.

Nutrition: Shape the Path

CHAPTER 4

Master Your Morning

*'Eat breakfast like a king, lunch like a prince
and dinner like a pauper.'*

— ADELLE DAVIS, author and nutritionist

J ack Dorsey, the CEO of tech giant Twitter, eats only one meal a day. In the late afternoon, he consumes one large feast, welcoming how a single meal per day frees up so much time for other things. Dorsey also regularly goes multiple days without eating, believing it provides him with a productivity edge. Is skipping breakfast really giving Dorsey a competitive edge? Or is it setting him up for major problems down the road? There are some key nuances to explore and meal timing is one of the most influential 'zeitgebers', or external cues, that impact your physiology and, indirectly, your ability to maintain a healthy weight.[1]

To Eat or Not to Eat?

Today, more and more people are skipping breakfast – as many as 25 per cent according to the latest polls.[2] Time restricted eating (TRE) is the term used to describe shrinking the 'window' in which you eat. For example, you might delay your breakfast or first meal until 11am or noon and stop eating at 6 or 7pm. You might have heard this type of dietary pattern being referred to as Intermittent Fasting, but this isn't quite right. Intermittent fasting (IF) is when you fast for two days per week, eating less than 500–800 calories on those days, and eating normally the remaining days of the week. Nevertheless, between TRE and IF, and many different variations in between, fasting is a popular option today.

But, does it help with weight loss? How about fighting off chronic conditions? In the complex and 'wicked' world of nutritional science, there are few clear-cut answers. But the research world has been abuzz with studies examining the benefits, and pitfalls, of eating (versus skipping) breakfast on weight loss and health. What should you do to reach PEAK40 health and performance? Let's dive into the research.

The Breakfast Research Timeline

In 2014, a randomized controlled trial of more than 300 overweight and obese adults investigated whether eating breakfast versus skipping breakfast over a 16-week period had any impact on weight loss. What did it reveal? Both groups had high compliance to their respective diets, yet breakfast consumption did not improve weight loss relative to breakfast skipping.[3] This added fuel to the 'skipping breakfast' fire – perhaps Jack Dorsey is on to something.

Over the next few years, the surge in popularity for TRE led the prestigious *British Medical Journal* to publish a review of 13 studies examining the effects of breakfast on weight loss.[4] Researchers wanted to put to the test the commonly held beliefs that skipping breakfast leads to more snacking later in the day and that eating breakfast helps to improve satiety for the rest of your day. What did they uncover? Scientists couldn't find consistent evidence that eating breakfast or skipping breakfast was superior for weight loss. Some people did lose weight, others did not. Some people improved their glucose and insulin levels (as well as appetite-controlling hormones like ghrelin or leptin), while others did not. However, researchers did find that people who eat breakfast tend to follow an array of healthy lifestyle choices: they exercise more regularly, they go to bed earlier, they consume more fibre and they're less likely to smoke or binge drink.[5] New science is starting to unpack with more precision the potential pitfalls of skipping breakfast and how eating the 'right' breakfast can lay the foundation for health and weight loss.

What Happens When You Skip Breakfast?

Let's circle back and look at the common traits of people who regularly skip breakfast. People who don't eat breakfast typically have higher HbA1c levels (a three-month average blood sugar control), higher diastolic blood pressure, higher triglycerides, higher uric acid levels (a marker of inflammation) and lower HDL-c levels.[6] Breakfast skippers are more likely to have a higher body weight, a greater risk of developing Type 2 diabetes and an increased prevalence of atherosclerosis.[7]

This connection between breakfast skipping and increased risk of atherosclerosis has been found to be *independent* of conventional heart disease risk factors in middle-aged adults (who do not suffer from any cardiovascular disease symptoms).[8] Breakfast skippers also have a higher risk of heart attack and stroke, regardless if they have a history of poor heart health.[9] People who skip breakfast often struggle with lifestyle behaviours as well. Breakfast skippers tend to stay up later and have poorer sleep quality. For example, sleep-deprived middle-aged adults show higher stress hormone levels, leading to greater arterial stiffness.[10] They also have a tendency towards lower mood and depressive symptoms.

If you're struggling with high blood glucose levels, it's important to note that skipping breakfast can amplify your glucose response to meals during the rest of the day and impair insulin secretion.[11] But it's important to remember, correlation isn't causation. Skipping breakfast isn't *causing* these outcomes.

If You're Lean and Active ...

New research on the impacts of eating breakfast for weight loss and health are uncovering some fascinating new insights. A few years ago, Dr Javier Gonzalez, PhD, and his team at Bath University in England compared how lean (defined as a BMI between 18.5–24.9kg/m^2) versus obese individuals responded to cutting out breakfast for an extended period of time. They recruited 49 individuals and, over a six-week period, instructed the breakfast group to consume at least 700 calories by 11am and a minimum of 50 per cent of those calories within two hours of getting up in the morning.[12] Participants could select various food options, however, most opted for the typical breakfast of cereal, toast and juice. Gonzalez assessed markers of body composition and cardiovascular and metabolic health before and after the intervention, as well as the activity of over 40 different genes and proteins. All this in an attempt to pinpoint scientifically what key physiological processes may be at play when eating, or skipping, breakfast.

How did breakfast impact the lean versus obese individuals? Eating breakfast resulted in a drop in fat-burning genes in lean individuals. This is not surprising because any time you consume food your body will put the brakes on body-fat breakdown and shift gears to burning the food you've eaten for fuel. Despite consuming significant calories for breakfast, the lean individuals burned off those calories throughout their typically very active day, offsetting the higher calories at breakfast. Things got interesting when they skipped breakfast. The lean individuals improved their capacity to burn body fat. In a fasted state, your body switches over to burning its fuel reserves (i.e. body fat) to fuel your day. If you are active and lean, some fasting in the morning can be beneficial to improve your ability to burn body fat.

Breakfast Helps Glucose Control If You're Overweight

How did the obese participants fair? Eating breakfast also resulted in a drop in fat-burning genes but, surprisingly, it decreased the activity of genes involved in insulin resistance. This was a novel twist. Eating breakfast in the obese group *improved* their ability to take up carbohydrates, a finding in step with previous research that showed breakfast consumption is associated with better glucose control in fat cells. This is a really important finding for obese and overweight individuals looking to improve glucose control and lose weight: eating breakfast helped (in a big way!). Another surprising finding in the obese group was that skipping breakfast increased the genes associated with inflammation, something not seen in the lean group. This has the potential to be problematic in the long-term for obese and overweight individuals, as chronic inflammation worsens glucose control. Skipping breakfast also worsens your blood glucose response to lunch – if you eat breakfast, your glucose tolerance at lunchtime improves, a phenomenon known as the 'second meal effect'.

In Summary

If you're obese or overweight, breakfast appears to be an important strategy for protecting against Type 2 diabetes and the subsequent adverse health effects of chronically high blood sugar levels. Of course, you need to pick the right breakfast. (More on this at the end of the chapter.)

If you're active and have a healthy body weight, you can choose from both options: skipping breakfast on specific days to support metabolic health (your body's ability to effectively burn body fat for fuel) and eating breakfast on the other days to support intense exercise and to avoid the pitfalls fasting can have on your daily energy expenditure and muscle mass.

This highlights the importance of individualized recommendations – context matters.

Does Skipping Breakfast Make You Move Less?

A morning meal might increase your daily calorie consumption, but there are two sides to the weight loss (energy balance) equation; energy in and energy out. Skipping breakfast definitely lowers your calorie intake. But skipping breakfast also has very subtle, yet highly significant, effects on your activity levels for the rest of the day. A recent study by Dr James Betts, PhD, at Bath University found that when you're in the fasted state in the morning, you end up expending less energy over the rest of the day.[13] That's right, it didn't matter if you were fit or obese, you ended up moving less. Something as trivial as fidgeting or blinking is, in fact, not so trivial; they can account for a significant amount of calories burned. In the long run, fewer calories burned per day through less physical activity, even through less fidgeting or daily movements, commonly leads to weight-loss plateaus.

Exercise First – A Better Strategy

Rather than skip breakfast, get some movement in before you eat breakfast. *When* you eat your food, whether before or after exercise, impacts how your body burns stored fat versus carbohydrate. The scientific term is nutrient-exercise timing: the effect that the food you eat has on your body's fuel of choice when exercising or even going about your day. The research of Dr Rob Edinburgh, PhD, investigated this question in a recent study and found that a single bout of exercise performed before (versus after) food intake increased the body's ability to break down stored body fat.[14] In short, if you exercise before you eat, it significantly improves your ability to burn stored body fat for fuel. Exercising before a meal also reduced insulin output after, meaning study participants were better able to tolerate carbohydrates.

Lift Weights before Breakfast

Edinburgh wasn't finished there. He also wanted to examine whether your muscles changed their preferred fuel source depending on whether your exercise was performed before (versus after) breakfast. In other words, does the timing of exercise also impact the fuel your muscles use? Edinburgh put study participants through a six-week training programme, before or after breakfast, to observe any possible changes to the fuel muscles preferred to use in the fasted versus fed state. Remarkably, they observed a two-fold increase in fat utilization by muscle tissue in the group training before breakfast. This is a really important point because when your muscles burn intramuscular triglycerides (the fat located in your muscle), it's a powerful signal to the body to improve insulin sensitivity as well. Impressively, this effect of muscle-burning intra-muscular fat for fuel was maintained throughout the six-week duration of the study when training was performed before carbohydrate ingestion.

Fasting and Exercise

Exercising in a fasted state benefits glucose control and insulin sensitivity without needing to increase the volume, intensity or perception of effort of your exercise.

- If you're trying to lose weight, improve glucose control or have a chronic health condition, exercising before breakfast is a terrific option, improving your body's ability to use fat for fuel, as well as improving your insulin sensitivity.
- If your schedule doesn't allow for it, similar effects can be had by exercising before lunch or dinner, provided you haven't snacked in the 3–4 hours prior to exercising.

It's Not Just Breakfast: The Pitfalls of Snacking

Here is the thing. You don't need a snack to get you from breakfast to lunch. Your body has more than enough fuel onboard to do the job. Not convinced? Even if you are 10 per cent body fat (aka – you can see abs), you would still have approximately 30,000 calories of energy stored as body fat. If you consider running a marathon requires 2,500–3,000 calories, that means you could run 10 marathons with no snacks or fuel (although, I wouldn't recommend it!). Snacking in mid-morning, for most of us, has just become a ritual or routine. This is problematic not just for the additional energy (calories) it brings, but because it sets up hunger cues for the long-term. Snack mid-morning regularly and, eventually, your brain will signal you to crave snacks mid-morning regularly.

Of course, if you eat the wrong type of breakfast, higher in simple sugars or processed carbs, it sends your blood sugar levels and energy skyrocketing up immediately after you eat. The problem is that by mid-morning, the blood sugar rollercoaster is thundering back down, leading to hypoglycemia and cravings. Your body can naturally control your glucose levels by burning body fat for fuel, you don't need to snack mid-morning to achieve this.

Why else is it important to ditch the mid-morning snack? Processed food consumption predicts excess calorie intake and weight gain and, in mid life, you're seemingly constantly surrounded by packaged foods at the office, during your commute and even at home.[15] This effect of processed food consumption and weight gain isn't a surprise to scientists; the best-known diet to fatten up mice for experimental studies is called the 'cafeteria' or 'supermarket' diet!

Table 4.1. Breakfast Options

Breakfast	Protein (g)
3 eggs + ½ avocado + ½ cup berries	20
Plain Greek yogurt (200g) + ½ cup raspberries + 2 tbsp crushed walnuts	24.3
Protein shake (30g) + ½ cup berries + water	31.2
Smoked salmon (100g) + cucumber + cherry tomatoes	23

Step 1: Master Your Morning

In the 'wicked' world of weight loss and fighting off chronic conditions, it's best to start with small solutions. Simple, clear and actionable first steps to get the ball rolling.

The first step to PEAK40 health and performance is to take back control of your morning, in order to set yourself up the right way for the day.

Here Is the *Master Your Morning* Plan:

1. Eat *at least* 20g protein with breakfast
2. Eliminate ultra-processed carbs
3. Ditch the snack between breakfast and lunch

Start with Protein

Achieving your ideal daily protein intake is a fundamental pillar for PEAK40 health and longevity. Breakfast is the meal of the day where people fail to consume an adequate amount of protein, so making a change here is a big opportunity for weight loss and health. Increasing your protein intake also increases your micronutrients intake in their most bioavailable form. Finally, eating protein 'costs' your body more energy to eat and digest, known as the thermic effect of food (TEF). What types of foods enable you to hit 20g protein (about the size of a deck of playing cards)? Table 4.1 gives a quick rundown.

This small change in your morning routine can have a big impact. For example, replacing your morning bowl of muesli or cereal for plain yogurt and berries reduces your carbohydrate and calorie intake by a whopping 60g and 240 calories, respectively. Ditch the mid-morning muffin or croissant from your local café and there is another significant reduction of approximately 40–50g and 160–200 calories, respectively. This is more than enough to trigger weight loss and better glucose, without changing your morning routine significantly (you still get to enjoy your coffee or tea!).

Don't worry, it's not a life sentence to low-carb breakfasts, just a targeted strategy to enhance your metabolic flexibility – your capacity to burn fat for fuel. (The leaner you are and the more your goals are performance-oriented, the higher your carb intake can be at breakfast. I'll discuss this more in Chapter 9.) It's also a great strategy to avoid the typical Western-style, calorie-dense breakfast of cereal, packaged breads, muffins and the like, which is associated with a lower mood later in the morning.[16] Finally, you can be creative: fill your plate with your preferred fruits and vegetables.

Exercise before Breakfast

Try exercising first thing in the morning to enhance the nutrient-exercise effects, if you're trying to lose weight or improve body composition. Whether it's walking, a run or lifting weights, you'll reap some of the additional benefits of insulin sensitivity and glucose control.

If you're already lean, fit and aiming for performance, your strategy will depend on the nature of your training session – low, moderate or intense – as well as your current training block and ultimate goal. (Refer to my first book *Peak* for more in-depth high-performance fuelling strategies.)

Make It a Habit

Getting into a routine, where your actions become habitual and automatic (like putting on your seatbelt), is the ultimate goal. Compliance is naturally highest at the start of the day, making the 'gap' between your current behaviour and this new *Master Your Morning* strategy quite small. You want to get to the point where you don't have to 'think' about what you're going to eat or how 'not to snack' in the morning, you just do it. Once you've *mastered your morning*, you've got one third of your day sorted.

Of course, with longer workdays, more evening leisure time and the advent of Netflix, we're consuming more calories than ever in the evening. Once you've *mastered your morning*, your next task is to *Own Your Night*.

CHAPTER 5

Own Your Night

'Not all who wander into the kitchen are lost.'
— UNKNOWN

Is that really Kyle Lowry? This was the essence of many Instagram comments in the summer of 2015 after a post went viral of a noticeably leaner Kyle Lowry, NBA all-star and starting point guard for the Toronto Raptors. His visual appearance was so dramatically different, it left many people around pro basketball wondering if it really was Kyle Lowry. It definitely was him. During the off-season, the stocky Lowry shed 6.8kg/15lb, trimming his body fat down to 5–6 per cent by dedicating himself to a new nutritional regime. Lowry was approaching 30, the mid life of a professional athlete, and he wanted to play at a high level into his mid to late 30s – unthought of a generation ago – and knew he needed to upgrade his nutrition game. He hired a performance nutritionist to plan and strategize his meal plans, and a professional chef to cook his food. Lowry was already an all-star but he wanted to be an NBA champion. His previous body weight and composition wouldn't allow his body to hold up to the rigours of the NBA. Interestingly, it wasn't just what Lowry's new chef and nutritionist *added* to his regime that made a difference, it's what they removed. Lowry had a history of struggling with late-night eating and it was a major roadblock to effective recovery and realizing his true potential.

When Treats Become Routine

The modern-day routine of longer working hours and eating later at night is having a significant impact on our health and waistline. After a long day at the office, you get home late and heat up a quick dinner, eat out or grab a takeaway, then collapse on the couch. It's not long before your brain craves a little snack – a glass of wine, piece of chocolate or small bowl of ice cream – while you watch the latest series on Netflix. The sugar hit provides your brain with a serotonin hit, that 'aah' feeling, after a long, busy day. It also provides a dopamine hit, the reward neurotransmitter that lets your brain know 'I like this' and reinforces the desire to engage in it again (and again). It's not long before your occasional treat becomes a habitual pattern. And when it does, your health, energy levels and waistline feel the effects. For Lowry, it was bags of Oreo cookies late at night after games. We all have our vices but, like Lowry, we also have the power to break the harmful pattern.

Eat More, Earlier

The pattern of eating 'small but often' – grazing throughout the day – is good advice gone wrong in today's ultra-processed food environment. Most people are eating for 15–18 hours per day, which simply gives us too much energy, and a big part of the problem is that most of the calories we consume are in the evening.

Chronic late-eating throws off your body's internal clocks and has been linked to obesity and metabolic disorders, such as pre-diabetes and diabetes.[1] The more calories you consume in the evening, the higher your BMI is likely to be. A recent study in overweight women looked into how weight gain is impacted by shifting more calories to the morning versus the end of the day. After three months, the women who consumed most of their calories at breakfast lost two and a half times more weight versus the women eating the majority at dinner. (Another reason why *Mastering Your Morning* is such a crucial piece of the puzzle.) Simply shifting more of your energy intake (i.e. calories) to earlier in the day is a big win for weight loss, blood sugars and biomarkers for health.[2] It also helps to improve your sleep quality. When you consume food in too close proximity to when you're going to sleep, it alters your melatonin output (the starter pistol for deep sleep) and thus delays and compromises your deep REM sleep.[3]

Late Eating Is the New Normal

In 2020, at the European and International Congress on Obesity, scientists from Ulster University in Northern Ireland presented data on the dietary habits of 1,200 UK adults who they had tracked from 2012–2017.[4] What did the data reveal? Over 40 per cent of all the calories consumed were *after* 6pm in the evening. It also highlighted that if you eat most of your calories in the evening, you are far more likely to follow a diet higher in ultra-processed foods, as well as drink more alcohol. Not surprisingly, they also found the later you stay up, the more likely you are to consume junk food and alcohol. (It seems very few people crave broccoli and Brussels sprouts late at night!) The researchers also revealed that individuals who consumed the most calories after 6pm were more likely to consume the *most calories* earlier in the day. It seems daytime behaviours trickle down to night-time as well. If you consumed the fewest calories after 6pm, however, you were more likely to consume the fewest calories earlier in the day. It seems we're quite consistent with our food intake.

The Impact of Eating Late

Nighttime eating, scientifically defined as having dinner close to or immediately before bed or having snacks after dinner, is linked to a two-fold greater risk of obesity and 1.5 times greater

Skipping Dinner Rather Than Breakfast

In Germany, researchers at the University of Hohenheim investigated whether skipping dinner versus breakfast impacted on how many calories you might burn in a day.[5] Study participants were assessed on a day when they skipped breakfast, a day when they ate three regular meals and a day when they skipped dinner. To ensure everything remained constant, the research team kept the calorie content of the meals and breakdown of carbohydrates, fat and protein the same on all three days. On days when breakfast or dinner was skipped, the other two meals made up the extra calories.

Blood samples were taken upon rising and throughout the day to assess for changes in blood glucose, insulin and hormone levels, as well as immune-system function. What did they find? Skipping dinner actually burned more than *double* the amount of calories (per day) compared to skipping breakfast. Not only that, skipping breakfast led to markedly higher glucose, insulin and inflammatory biomarkers.

Skipping breakfast isn't just a North American or European problem. In Japan, researchers examined the same question and found study participants who skipped breakfast consumed far more calories later in the day. Specifically, they ate late dinners, ate more ready-made meals (rather than cooking) and succumbed to more late-night snacking.[6] (Sounds familiar, right?) This isn't to suggest you should skip dinner, but it can be an effective, evidence-based strategy to overcome weight-loss plateaus when applied on a few nights per week, for a specific period of time.

risk of dyslipidaemia.[7] This relationship is true even after correcting for age, physical activity and smoking and alcohol intake.

Late-night eating is also connected to a 55 per cent higher risk of heart disease compared to an earlier dinner time.[8] A recent study found eating at night was positively associated with a higher BMI in middle-aged participants, as well as worsening of arterial stiffness, leading to higher blood pressure.[9] Researchers concluded that shifting calorie intake to earlier in the day would help to offset these effects.

When late-night eating is made up of calorie-dense, nutrient-poor processed foods, it leads to a big bump in glucose and fatty acid levels in the bloodstream, the rush of sugar and fat kicking up free radical damage and inflammation, damaging and stiffening the inner lining of your arteries.[10] The more you engage in night eating or late-night snacking, the more likely you are to smoke, consume alcohol and be sedentary. It can also worsen your glucose response to breakfast the next morning. For most people, the poor lifestyle choices come first, followed by the late-night snacking. In short, if you want to achieve PEAK40 health and performance in mid life, it's time to tackle late-night eating.

Working against Our Bodies

Modern science has uncovered that your glucose tolerance is best in the morning, after an overnight fast, and becomes poorer in the evening and closer to bedtime. Our circadian rhythms, linked to the light and dark cycles of the day, are deeply hard-wired into our body's operating system after millions of years of evolution. When you eat late at night, you disrupt the body's internal clocks that control your blood glucose levels, adrenaline and stress hormone cortisol output, as well as key appetite regulating hormones.[11] From an evolutionary perspective, this makes sense; it was difficult to snack past sundown for hundreds of thousands of years and our genes still operate on this evolutionary model.

Interestingly, a primary tenet of Traditional Chinese Medicine (TCM), which dates back over 3,000 years, is that the body's response to food varies at different times of the day. Experts believe this effect is due to the natural daily rhythms of the beta-cells of your pancreas and how well your body tissues can take up insulin as the day grows long. Eating too close to bedtime forces your pancreas, gut and fat tissues to 'turn on' and process the ingested meal, at a time when your body is attempting to ramp down activity.[12] Your circadian rhythms are influenced by a number of factors: light exposure, activity, timing of food intake and caffeine.

Having a plan for how you start your day (*Master Your Morning*) and finish the day (*Own Your Night*), where things typically go wrong, are essential elements to PEAK40 health and performance. Kyle Lowry had a game plan for his nutrition and three years after making significant changes to his diet and lifestyle regime, Lowry surpassed his goal of simply making it to the NBA

Step 2: Own Your Night

If you create a clear path for the Elephant to follow, it becomes much easier to keep it moving forwards in the desired direction. This is where having rules about what days you can snack, and which days you cannot, is very important. You don't want to be making food decisions while you're sitting on the couch at 9 or 10pm after a long day. You need a game plan ahead of time to keep the Elephant on track. Simple, actionable steps you can implement and feel the difference quickly.

Here Is the *Own Your Night* Plan:

1. Eat dinner no later than 8pm – *i.e. no food after 8pm (hard rule), preferably closer to 6–7pm (if possible, for better results)*
2. Avoid late snacking *for at least 5 nights per week (weekends open)*
    Instead:
    - sip herbal tea (caffeine-free)
    - take a warm bath or hot shower
    - perform light stretching
    - go to a quiet room in the house and read

If you can commit to eating dinner no later than 8pm, refrain from snacking five nights per week and make a weekend 'treat' truly a treat, you'll lay another important pillar to PEAK40 health and performance in mid life.

finals. In 2019, he played a pivotal role in leading the Toronto Raptors to their first ever NBA championship. It wasn't just his dedication to his basketball craft that allowed him to achieve his PEAK performance, it was his dedication to establishing high-performance habits with his nutrition and lifestyle.

CHAPTER 6

Set Your Protein

'I don't believe in philosophies. I believe in fundamentals.'
— JACK NICKLAUS, golfer

In 2011, Rory McIlroy was standing on the 10th tee at Augusta National Golf Club in Georgia, leading the Masters tournament and in search of his first major championship win. Rory's golf swing, short game and putting stroke were all seemingly dialled in and he was only nine holes away from a lifelong dream. Unfortunately, Rory's dream of winning the Masters evaporated with one bad swing, a snap hook out of bounds off the 10th tee, and he staggered to the clubhouse with a final round score of 80. McIlroy's body language told the whole story: head down, dragging his feet and muttering to himself as he walked off the last green, an embarrassing eight over par for the day. Golf is an incredibly challenging game, just when you think you've got it figured out, it throws you for a loop (even the best in the world). What did Rory McIlroy do after his collapse at the Masters? Change his swing? Change his clubs? Nope. He went to work on the practice tee, spending more hours working on the fundamentals of grip, stance and alignment, so next time he was under pressure he would have the habits required to succeed. Mastery is only achieved when you're an expert in the fundamentals. In golf, moments of failure are inevitable, just like when you're trying to lose weight. Roadblocks are inevitable; they're a normal part of the learning process. What lessons can you learn from world-class performers like McIlroy? If you're struggling with weight gain, you don't need to pivot to a completely new diet or exercise regime, you simply need to go back to the basics and improve your fundamentals. Now that you've learned how to *Master Your Morning* and *Own Your Night*, it's time to *Set Your Protein*.

Protein is a critical keystone to support your performance and health goals and it provides the foundation to *Master Your Morning*, *Own Your Night* and everything that comes in between. Once you've determined your optimal protein intake (and it becomes a habit), it frees up more time and headspace to address the rest of your diet and integrate other key behaviour changes.

Why is protein so essential for your body? Proteins are the building blocks of life. They build everything, from your red blood cells that provide oxygen to your cells, and hormones that support energy and satiety, to immune cells that fight off bacteria, neurotransmitters that influence emotions and thoughts, and muscles that support longevity. If you're the house, proteins are the bricks. The busier, more active and more stressed you are, the more bricks your body needs to maintain health. In mid life, this can easily catch up to you.

Back to Basics – Protein 101

Regardless of whether you eat a chicken breast, a salmon fillet or a handful of almonds, the proteins you consume are broken down in your gut to their simplest form: the individual amino acids. There are 20 basic amino acids which, like Lego bricks, act as the building blocks for all the proteins in the body. They are made up of only four things: oxygen, hydrogen, carbon and nitrogen elements.

It's Not about Plant vs. Animal

Scroll through your social media feed and you'll quickly run into a plethora of 'plant-based' versus 'animal-based' debates raging online. Rather than believing the false dichotomy of having to choose between plant or animal, why not do both? (Or think of it as a continuum and find where you prefer to be.) Let's start with why animal proteins are key for health.

Unpacking Animal Protein

Milk and eggs are considered the gold standard for protein quality of any food by nutritional scientists. Why? Animal proteins contain all the essential amino acids required for life, in a much more bioavailable form (i.e. easier to digest and utilize) compared to plant-based foods. Animal protein is also the richest source of leucine (a key essential amino acid responsible for triggering muscle growth and repair) and creatine (a high-energy protein), both of which are critically important when it comes to building lean muscle mass. Protein is also tremendously nutrient dense, containing a treasure trove of essential vitamins and minerals and healthy fats. For example, 30 per cent of the fatty acid content of conventional red meat is oleic acid (aka – olive oil), which has been championed in the Mediterranean diet for its cholesterol-lowering effect and connection to reduced risk of blood pressure and stroke.[1] Meat gets an undeserved bad rap when it comes to health, considering it's a group 1 NOVA food, raw or minimally processed. It's the processed burgers and fast-food hot dogs you need to limit.

However, just because animal proteins are health-giving, doesn't mean you should *only* eat meat. (This is particularly true when it comes to factory-farmed animals. The harmful impacts of factory farming are clear and the practice should be abolished. It harms the animal, it harms the environment and it yields lower quality food.)

Variety Is Key for Plant Protein

Plant-based proteins have a lot to offer, including an abundance of micronutrients, as well as the added bonuses of high fibre and antioxidant contents. From a scientific perspective, vegetable

Mix Up Your Veg Protein

Vegetarians and vegans should obtain a mix of vegetable protein sources at every meal. In general, grains are deficient in the amino acid lysine and beans are low in methionine. By combining two of the following three food groups, you can achieve sufficient levels of all the essential amino acids:

- beans and pulses
- grains
- nuts and seeds

proteins are considered inferior to animal proteins because they are typically deficient in one of the essential amino acids and are absorbed at only 70 per cent efficiency when compared to animal sources. Therefore, if you follow a strict plant-based or vegan diet, you may be short of the full complement of essential amino acids necessary to achieve good health. Of course, you can easily correct for these limitations by increasing your intake of plant-based proteins. See Table 6.1, page 73, for a comprehensive list (or go to DrBubbs.com/PEAK40 to download a full list of protein options).

Common Concerns about a Higher Protein Intake

A few questions often emerge when you ask someone to increase their protein intake. First, will it be harmful (rather than beneficial) to health and ramp up the risk for heart disease, Type 2 diabetes or various cancers?

The primary concern in medical circles is around the saturated fat content of animal protein, primarily red meat, dairy and eggs. The *American Heart Association* declared in 2015 that 'cholesterol is not a nutrient of concern for overconsumption', which means you can strike that one off the list. However, saturated fat intake is still a topic of much debate.[2]

The myth that a higher protein intake is harmful to your kidneys still persists in the media and some medical circles. Research conducted by Dr Jose Antonio, PhD, showed no adverse effects on kidney function when a very high protein intake of 3 grams of protein per kilogram of bodyweight per day (3g/kg/day), almost triple the minimum I recommend here, was consumed for an entire year.[3] Protein expert Stuart Phillips, PhD, sums up the research succinctly, 'high protein intake is not damaging to healthy kidneys.'[4]

The challenge in clinical practice is that these myths dissuade people from achieving the desired level of protein intake – a major hurdle when trying to lose weight or improve health. Understanding the nuances is part of the problem. You don't just eat 'saturated fats', you eat beef and the tens of thousands of nutrients it contains. The challenge with solving any complex problem in 'wicked' environments is the high degree of uncertainty and ambiguity. Let's review some new research which teases out the difference between processed and unprocessed red meat.

Unprocessed vs. Processed Red Meat: Diabetes and Heart Health

A major shortcoming of public health recommendations is that they fail to distinguish between processed meat, such as hot dogs, sausages, bacon and the like, and unprocessed 'red meat', like a grass-fed steak or pastured-fed lamb. There is a massively important distinction, even for those who are not meat-centric. New research confirms it's the intake of *processed meat* that has been associated with an increased risk of heart disease and not the consumption of *unprocessed* red meat.[5] And recent large meta-analysis found processed meat consumption increases the risk of Type 2 diabetes as well.[6] Processed meats are typically deep fried and much higher in calories, via fat or added sugars, compared to natural, minimally processed meats. Not convinced yet? The aforementioned meta-analysis in Type 2 diabetics found no such association with unprocessed red meat and diabetes. The quality of what you eat matters. The battle isn't plant versus animal; it's processed versus unprocessed.

What about heart health? New research of randomized control trials reveals 'very low' to 'low' quality of evidence supporting the claim *unprocessed or minimally processed* red meat has adverse effects on heart and metabolic health.[7]

Red meat is also an incredibly nutrient-dense food; a complete source of protein, high in essential vitamins and minerals (including highly absorbable iron), along with modest amounts of omega-3 in grass-fed varieties.[8] Whether you choose to include red meat in your diet is entirely up to you. Just don't eliminate it from your diet because you believe, or have been told, it's unhealthy. In my experience working with elite performers across many professions, including some red meat goes a long way to achieving PEAK40 health and performance.

A Good Egg

Eggs are another food often seen in scare-mongering headlines, such as this one stating, 'Eating just one egg a day increases your risk of developing Type 2 diabetes by 60 per cent, according to a new study.'[9] Unfortunately, this is just bad science. First, correlation is not causation. Just because two things are happening at the same time, doesn't mean one is *causing* the other. But, more importantly, the researchers in the aforementioned egg study didn't even control for the rest of the subject's intake of toast, cereal, hash browns, sugar, etc. In 2020, a comprehensive review in the *American Journal of Clinical Nutrition* of more than 177,000 people from 50 different countries, led a panel of expert researchers from around the world to conclude 'no significant associations between egg intake and blood lipids, mortality or major CVD events'.[10]

More Protein = More Micronutrients

Protein also contains a wealth of micronutrients. When you increase your protein intake, you also dramatically increase your vitamin and mineral intake as well, which enhances the overall quality of your diet.[11]

This is especially important when you consider the recent *Dietary Guidelines for Americans,* which identified numerous micronutrients that are under-consumed and considered insufficient in our diets today, including calcium, choline (vitamin B4), folate, iron, magnesium, water-soluble vitamins B12 and C, and fat-soluble vitamins A, D, E and K.[12] These essential micronutrients play key roles in supporting your blood pressure and bone and heart health, and a lower intake can seriously hinder your ability to push yourself and perform in training.[13]

Eating the right amount of protein, for you, is a fundamental pillar to preventing these deficiencies and supporting overall health. A recent review study found, 'habitually consuming high-protein diets ... was associated with better overall diet quality scores in both males and females.'[14] Even more compelling, this effect was independent of fruit and vegetable intake. Of course, why not do both? Enhance your protein intake and eat a lot of veggies and fruit! To sum up, the research clearly shows if you eat more real-food protein sources, you'll ramp up your intake of key micronutrients.[15]

More Protein Does Not Make You Fat

Protein intake plays a pivotal role when it comes to weight loss, not only because it helps to build and maintain lean muscle, improves satiety and costs your body more calories just to digest it, but it's also virtually impossible to convert into body fat. A recent study investigated how dramatically over-feeding protein to bodybuilders (4.4g/kg/per day) might impact their fat gain. The total calories from the excess protein equalled 800 calories per day and incredibly did not lead to any changes in fat mass.[16] If you were to overeat 800 calories from carbohydrates or fats, you would certainly add fat mass. In short, protein helps improve body composition in a number of ways and is virtually impossible to convert into body fat (big wins!).

Like golf, nutrition isn't about how well you do on your best days, but rather limiting the damage on your bad days. Two months after his disappointing finish at the Masters in 2011, Rory Mc-Ilroy destroyed the competition at the US Open, winning his first major championship by an incredible 8-shot margin. When things go wrong, it's easy (and natural) to think you're a long way off target. The reality is, you're likely to be only a few degrees off course. Rory doubled down on trusting the process, knowing the results would come. Now, it's time for you to do the same.

Step 3: Set Your Protein

Currently, the recommended dietary allowance (RDA) for protein is 0.8g/kg/per day. However, protein experts around the world are finding in their research that this amount is insufficient to support health and longevity.

The total amount of protein you should aim to eat each day is a *minimum* of 1.2g/kg/per day to achieve PEAK40 health and performance.

> For example, if you weigh 100kg (220lb), this would mean 120g protein per day. If you weigh 70kg (154lb), this would be 84g protein daily.

How much protein is this? Well, 20g is approximately the size of a deck of playing cards. Or, if you prefer another estimate, you can use your hand size. For women, the size and thickness of your palm is about 20–30g protein and for men it is approximately 30–40g.

The benefits of achieving this protein intake isn't just about your goals in your 40s, it's also about setting you up for PEAK health in your 50s, 60s and beyond! As you pass the age of 60, loss of muscle mass and bone density become serious concerns and new research shows older adults require more protein to reach the same muscle protein synthesis (MPS) threshold, compared to younger individuals.[17] Achieving the 1.2g/kg/per day protein target today will help you to maintain your muscle and bone health tomorrow.

Here Is Your *Set Your Protein* Plan

Total Protein: Achieve at least 1.2g/kg/per day of protein.

Aim for *at least* 20g high-quality protein at each meal. Most people fail to hit this target at breakfast, so that is a big opportunity to upgrade how you start your day (see Table 4.1, page 51).

Trying to lose weight or gain muscle? Aim for 1.6g/kg/per day. If adding more muscle and getting leaner is your primary goal, increasing your intake a little does yield significant benefits. Protein expert Dr Robert Morton, PhD, from McMaster University in Canada has shown that the sweet spot for protein intake is approximately 1.6g/kg/per day to maximize benefits for muscle mass and body composition.[18] If you bump up your intake to this level, you will likely see noticeable gains.[19]

If you're a plant-based eater, reaching 1.6g/kg/per day is also an important target. The benefits are the same whether the protein comes via plant or animal sources, once you hit this figure. A big win if you follow a strict plant-based diet.

Timing of Protein: Divide your protein intake over three to four meals daily.

Once you've set your protein intake, your next goal is protein timing. This simply means spreading out your protein intake evenly throughout the day. Ideally, this would be over three to four 'meals' per day (i.e. breakfast, lunch, an optional afternoon snack and dinner). If

Table 6.1. Protein Sources

Red Meat	Protein (g)	Fish	Protein (g)
Sirloin steak	27	Mackerel	19
Ribeye	24	Salmon	20
Ground beef	26	Anchovies	29
Lamb	25	Sardines	25
Venison	30	Herring	25
Bison	26	Tuna	30
Oxtail	8	Haddock	24
Poultry/Fowl	**Protein (g)**	**Seafood**	**Protein (g)**
Chicken thighs	24	Oysters	24
Chicken breast	30	Mussels	24
Turkey breast	29	Scallops	20
Duck breast	29	Shrimp	24
Dairy/Eggs	**Protein (g)**	Clams	26
Eggs (×2)	12	**Plant Proteins**	**Protein (g)**
Milk (250ml)	8	Soy yogurt	5
Plain yogurt	10	Soy milk (250ml)	8
Cottage cheese	11	Lentils	9
Ricotta	11	Beans	9
Parmesan (2 tbsp)	4	Edamame	11

Note: All protein amounts listed above are based on 100g (3.5oz) serving, unless otherwise stated.

you eat three square meals per day, then you'll need to hit your protein total in three meals.

For most people, I recommend a protein-based snack, such as yogurt, milk or soy milk, or a protein supplement in the afternoon, to equal four meals, to make it a little easier to achieve your protein target, as well as to help fight off cravings and keep energy levels stable.

Another benefit of dividing your protein intake evenly over the course of the day is that it means you don't need to rush home to drink your protein shake after exercise.

But, is there a scenario where protein timing really does matter? If you're training in a fasted state or if you're training multiple times in one day, then consuming protein directly after exercise is very helpful.[20]

Types of Protein: Eat a wide variety of animal and plant protein sources.

The last consideration when it comes to eating protein is 'type'. Consuming a wide variety of different protein sources leads to the consumption of a greater array of micronutrients. Interestingly, individuals who consume a higher protein intake generally consume more vegetables, more dark leafy greens, more legumes, more whole grains, more dairy and fewer empty calories (i.e. ultra-processed foods), compared to the general population.[21]

Table 6.1 contains a comprehensive list of protein types to choose from. Do your best to select proteins from each category to achieve a diverse intake.

CHAPTER 7

Turn the Dial on Carbs

'It's not that I'm so smart, it's just that I stay with problems longer.'
— ALBERT EINSTEIN, theoretical physicist

Kelly Holmes is a world-class middle-distance runner, bronze medal winner at the 2000 Sydney Olympics in the 800m event and the British record holder for the 600, 800 and 1,000 metres. Middle-distance running is a gruelling sport; the distances are short enough to require all out efforts, but long enough to require the stamina to tolerate a high degree of pain and discomfort. Success wasn't a straight line for Holmes. She started her athletic career at the age of 12, inspired by Olympians at the 1980 Olympic Games, and won the English Schools 1,500-metre championship two years later. But her athletics career ended abruptly, as she left school early to work. Then, at the age of 18, she decided to join the Army and her passion for exercise was re-ignited; first, as a basic physical training instructor, then as British Army judo champion, and later competing against the men in the 1,500-metre race (she was too fast for the other women). Fast forward to 2003 and Holmes was training in France in preparation for the 2004 Olympics when she suffered a significant leg injury – a devastating blow in the lead up to an Olympic year. When confronted with a complex problem you have two options: continue to press on (and figure out a solution), or give up. Holmes was not a quitter. She continued to move forward, re-assessing all areas of her health and putting a plan together to overcome the obstacles in her way en route to the 2004 Olympics. Would it be enough? She would need to trust the process.

Solving complex problems in 'wicked' domains takes time. Weight loss isn't linear, nor is improving high blood pressure or low mood. You must be patient and you must observe. Failure or setbacks provide you with the opportunity to learn about yourself, to tinker and troubleshoot, to uncover the root causes of *why* you're not achieving your health and performance goals. There is no magic bullet. Consistency and effort are the secrets to success, and you'll need them to navigate the nuances of how to adjust your carbohydrate intake to achieve your PEAK40 health and performance goals.

The Big Picture: They Are Not All Equal

Let's talk carbohydrates. The scientific term for carbohydrates is saccharides. They can be divided into three general groups: monosaccharides, disaccharides and polysaccharides. Monosaccharides are the simplest form of carbohydrate, absorbed more rapidly into the bloodstream and consisting of only one sugar. They typically have a sweet taste and examples include glucose, fructose (which is found primarily in fruit), natural sweeteners (such as honey) and processed sweeteners (such as high-fructose corn syrup [HFCS]). Disaccharides, made up of two monosaccharide sugars linked together, are also considered simple sugars and are absorbed quickly into the bloodstream. For example, sucrose or table sugar is a disaccharide formed when one fructose molecule is linked to one glucose molecule. Other examples of disaccharides include those naturally found in milk, called lactose, and maltose, which is found in cereals, pasta and beer. Lastly, polysaccharides are complex carbohydrate molecules, named so because they contain many monosaccharide units linked together, like branches of a tree. Complex carbs are broken down slowly and steadily into glucose subunits to fuel activity or exercise and can be stored as glycogen. The fibre contained in complex carbs helps to slow the release of the glucose subunits, a major reason why processed 'white' versions are absorbed much more quickly than whole food varieties. Examples of polysaccharide-rich foods include rice, potatoes, grains, root vegetables, tubers (vegetables that grow below ground) and corn, all of which have been dietary staples in various traditional populations across the globe.

You can think of carbohydrates like the fuel you put in your car's tank. The more you drive, the more fuel you need. The less you drive, the less fuel you need. The same goes for carbs; the more you move, the more carbohydrates you can likely tolerate in your diet. The less you move, you'll likely benefit with fewer. For example, an 80kg/176lb elite basketball player requires 400g carbohydrates a day during competition, while a 100kg/220lb American football lineman needs 500–600g, and a 70kg/154lb professional cyclist requires 700–800g (the equivalent of about 10–12 plates of cooked pasta!). Athletes fuel based on the demands of the work required. If they are training hard and expending this many calories, simple sugars can play a key role in providing enough fuel in the tank to train at high intensity and recover effectively. (It's hard to hit these totals with rice and spaghetti alone.)

Of course, if you change the context and focus on the general population, the entire equation gets flipped on its head. If humans have been eating complex carbs for thousands of years, yet the global obesity epidemic is only 40 years old, are whole food carbohydrates *really* the problem? No, of course not. Too many simple sugars or carbohydrates, i.e. too many calories, when you're not as active, can quickly lead to an excess of energy, raising your blood glucose levels, blood pressure, inflammation and body weight.[1]

The Problem with Processed Carbs

The problem is that there is simply too much energy in the modern diet and that 'extra energy' is either coming from carbs and/or fats, usually through ultra-processed, convenience snack foods and tasty treats. (Remember that protein is virtually impossible to convert into fat when consumed in excess.)

It's not just the blood sugar highs and lows that are problematic; too many simple sugars and processed carbohydrates also raise your blood saturated fatty acid levels, that pesky biomarker connected to poor health outcomes (and erroneously attributed to red meat, dairy and egg intake). If your blood levels of circulating saturated fatty acids are high, you are at higher risk of poor metabolic health, obesity, diabetes, heart attack and mortality.[2] Multiple studies show a direct link between excess carbohydrate intake from processed foods and high levels of saturated fatty acids (e.g. palmitoleic acid) in the blood that occur independent of saturated fat intake.[3] Even if you're not diabetic, high saturated fatty acid levels in the blood are highly problematic.[4]

What's Right for You?

The final step to PEAK40 nutrition is to *Turn the Dial* on (adjust) your carbohydrate (and fat) intake. Like knobs on a DJ mixing deck, you can turn down (or turn up) your carb and/or fat intake to suit your goals and the demands of your day.

Are you fit and physically active? You are likely to require a greater amount of carbohydrates overall and/or at certain meals of the day (before or after training).

Are you trying to lose 9kg/20lb and improve your blood glucose control? If so, then reducing carbohydrate intake (particularly before exercise) is the better option in the short-term.

As you can see, context matters. Where should you start to direct your focus? Let's examine three key areas:

- Cruciferous veggies
- Dietary nitrates
- Whole food carbs

Cruciferous Veggies

Getting enough vegetables in your diet is a fundamental piece of the PEAK40 puzzle. Vegetables bring the antioxidants, vitamins, minerals and fibre needed to fight off CVD, diabetes, cancer and other chronic conditions that take root in mid life.[5] Certain vegetables pack a little more healthful punch than others and cruciferous vegetables are at the top of the list.

Cruciferous vegetables, such as asparagus, broccoli, Brussels sprouts, kale, cabbage and the like (see Table 7.1), contain bioactive compounds, like sulphur, and contain glucosinolates and S-methylcysteine sulfoxide, flavonoids, anthocyanins, carotenoids and more, that exert powerful beneficial effects. For example, cruciferous veggies protect your heart and arteries by reducing LDL-c levels, combating free radical damage and ramping up glutathione activity (the body's all-star antioxidant).[6] The more cruciferous veggies you include in your diet, the less likely you are to develop diabetes.[7] The more cruciferous vegetables you include in your diet, the less likely you are to be obese in mid life.[8] And, finally, the more cruciferous veggies you include in your diet, the better your protection against cognitive decline and Alzheimer's.[9]

Cruciferous veggies are also a great source of fibre, which helps to keep your glucose levels stable, your gut bacteria diverse and prevent chronic conditions. In fact, the more fibre you eat, the lower your risk of mortality from any cause.[10] You may have already heard about many of the benefits of cruciferous vegetables,

Table 7.1. Cruciferous Vegetables

Broccoli and Its Cousins	Leafy Greens	Root Vegetables
Broccoli	Kale	Radishes
Brussels sprouts	Pak choy or Bok choy	Swede/Rutabaga
Cauliflower	Swiss chard	Turnips
Green cabbage	Collard greens	
Red cabbage	Mustard greens	
	Watercress	

but to master the fundamentals means upgrading your *application* of the knowledge. Aim to consume one serving per day of cooked cruciferous vegetables. Table 7.1 shows a brief list of commonly found cruciferous vegetables to include in your diet.

Dietary Nitrates

Green leafy vegetables, like rocket/arugula, spinach, lettuce and pak choy or bok choy, are among the most cardioprotective vegetables for keeping arteries strong and healthy.[11] What makes these veggies so special? They contain very high amounts of dietary nitrates, shown to reduce high blood pressure in both the short-term and the long-term.[12] Dietary nitrates are key nutrients that help to deliver more oxygen to your tissues to support health, lower high blood pressure and even exercise performance. In patients with chronic ischemia – lack of blood flow to the heart – increasing dietary nitrate consumption has been shown to improve revascularization, helping to restore better blood flow to the heart. That's the power of nitrate-rich vegetables. The problem is, the general population just doesn't consume enough of them.[13]

How Many Dietary Nitrates Should You Aim to Consume Daily?

The average intake of dietary nitrates is around 100mg per day. However, this can vary from as low as 20mg to as high as 400mg in people who consume a lot of vegetables.[14] Research suggests 400mg per day is a great target; enough to increase blood nitrate levels and support vascular health. See Table 7.2 for a list of high-nitrate vegetables (or go to DrBubbs.com /PEAK40 to download a full list of nitrate-rich foods).

Table 7.2. High-Nitrate Vegetables

Vegetable	Nitrates (mg/100g)
Rocket/Arugula	480
Celery	250
Spinach	250
Watercress	250
Beetroot / Beet juice	250
Beetroot/Beets	110–179
Chinese cabbage	160
Swiss chard	147
Mustard greens	116
Pak choy or Bok choy	100
Turnips	100
Parsley	100
Carrots	90

Step 4: Turn the Dial on Your Carb Intake

A common mistake people make is feeling that they need to adopt a 100 per cent low-carb or low-fat dietary strategy. You don't. Rather than committing to a strict adherence to a specific dietary strategy, you can do what the best athletes and Olympians do – adjust your intake based on the demands of your day. In my first book, *Peak: The New Science of Athletic Performance That Is Revolutionizing Sports*, I dive into the concept of carbohydrate periodization used by elite endurance and team sport nutritionists and staff – varying your meals between low, moderate and high carb.

I'll provide you with some general carbohydrate targets to get started but, remember, it will take some time to dial in the right combination for you. Be patient. How many carbohydrates should *you* eat in a day?

Your Carb Intake Plan

If you're struggling with high blood pressure, blood
    sugar levels or pre-diabetes and are looking to lose
    10kg (22lb) or more, then a good place to start is
    between 0.5–1.0g/kg/per day of carbohydrates.
If moderate weight loss of between around 5–10kg
    (11–22lb) is your goal, consider 0.5–1.5g/kg/per day.
If you are aiming for weight loss of less than 5kg
    (12lb), try between 0.5–2.0g/kg/per day. Notice

the lower end stays the same, while the upper threshold increases the fitter and healthier you are. If you're very fit or athletic (i.e. you can see abs), you may require up to 3–3.5g/kg/per day, or more depending on your sport and goals.

Carb Timing

- Eat more carbs earlier in the day; consume fewer later in the evening.
- Prioritize carb intake around exercise or activity – ideally, after exercising, if you are aiming for weight loss; consume fewer when sedentary.
- If consuming simple sugars, immediately before exercise (within 15 minutes), during exercise, or immediately after is best (limit if weight loss is your primary goal).
- Avoid simple carbs before bed.

Carb Type

- Whole foods (e.g. the ingredient list has one word)

How can you adjust your carb intake up or down? My preferred strategies with clients are *carb swaps* and *ratchet carbs*.

Strategy A: Carb Swaps

The amount of carbohydrates can vary significantly from one food to another. Carbohydrate sources like rice and pasta are more carbohydrate dense — they contain a greater amount of carbohydrates by volume (per cup) than other sources, such as white potatoes or beetroot/beets.

For example, one cup of cooked carrots has approximately 12g carbohydrates (48 calories), while the same serving size of boiled potatoes has double at 24g (96 calories) and the equivalent serving of cooked rice or pasta has 3.5 times more than carrots at 40 and 45g carbs (160 and 180 calories), respectively. By swapping out rice for roasted carrots, you can reduce your carb and calorie intake by 33g and 132 calories, respectively, without changing the amount of food on your plate.

Again, this doesn't make rice and pasta 'bad' and carrots 'good'. Pasta is a great carb to include for athletes who are training hard and looking to build lean muscle, or for high-level endurance athletes logging a lot of miles every day. But it does contain a high density of carbohydrates, so if you're mainly at your desk all day, it's not the best choice.

Strategy B: Ratchet Carbs

The second simple tool I use with clients is to ratchet up, or ratchet down, your carb intake at meals. Thus, it's not just the type of carb you can adjust, you can also adjust your portion sizes.

Don't think of this strategy as 'portion control', as that term suggests you lack the willpower to control

Table 7.3. Carbohydrate Sources

Roots and Tubers	Carbs (g)	Fruit	Carbs (g)
Turnips	8	Strawberries	12
Swede/Rutabaga	11	Blackberries	14
Carrots	12	Raspberries	15
Beetroot/Beets	13	Pineapple	20
White potatoes	24	Blueberries	21
Parsnips	24	Apple	25
Sweet potatoes	27	Pear	27
Yams	42	Banana	30
Plantains	47	**Pseudo-Cereals**	**Carbs (g)**
Yucca/Cassava	51	Buckwheat	24
Cereal Grains	**Carbs (g)**	Quinoa	42
Oats	25	Amaranth	46
Bread (2 slices)	28	**Dried Fruit**	**Carbs (g)**
Millet	41	Apricots (×6)	26
Wholewheat pasta	45	Figs (×4)	26
		Raisins (¼ cup)	32
White rice	52	Cranberries (¼ cup)	33
Brown rice	45	Medjool dates	36

Note: All carbohydrate amounts listed above are per cup, unless otherwise stated.

your food choices (remember, willpower is a finite resource). Ratcheting carbs means precisely that: strategically increasing or decreasing the amount you consume at meals (to achieve your desired goal). See Table 7.3 for a comprehensive list of carbohydrate choices and how many grams of carbohydrate they contain per cup. Having an idea of how many carbs are in your typical portion is crucial for establishing a baseline. From there, you can *ratchet down* or *ratchet up* as needed. But, fear not, this isn't going to turn into measuring every piece of food that goes into your mouth. Rather, it accomplishes a very important task; it provides you with a visual cue for how much to eat.

Whole Food (Minimally Processed) Carbs

Carbohydrates from whole food sources are very nutrient dense, providing the vitamins, minerals, antioxidants and fibre to support your best health. It's important to include a variety of different carbohydrate types in your diet to ensure you maximize your nutrient density.

Roots and tuberous vegetables, such as sweet potatoes, yams, yucca (cassava), plantains, carrots, beetroot/beets, parsnips, turnips and swede/rutabaga, have been staple foods for people in Africa, Asia and Latin America for centuries. They provide raw/minimally processed carbohydrate options loaded with vitamins, minerals and antioxidants.

Reducing Carbs for Weight Loss

How many carbs should you aim to reduce? In order to trigger weight loss, you're looking to trim about 250–400 calories per day from your meals. This equals about 70–100g of carbohydrates. If your diet consists of the typical 300+ grams per day, it should be quite straightforward to trim your intake.

- For example, ditch the banana and muesli on your yogurt for breakfast in favour of berries and you'll trim 60–80g carbs (240–320 calories).
- Swapping a standard portion of rice for white potatoes at dinner reduces your carb intake from 70g to 40g. The difference of 30g is equal to a reduction of 120 calories.

Total reduction: 90–110g (360–440 calories)

Pseudo-cereals are broad-leaved plants (non-grasses), they are naturally gluten-free and can be used in a similar way to traditional grains. Examples of pseudo-cereals include quinoa, amaranth and buckwheat (note: although it contains 'wheat' in its name, buckwheat is a broad-leaved plant and not a grass related to wheat).

Lastly, traditional cereal grains, such as white, brown and wild rice varieties, oats, millet, as well as freshly made sourdough (as opposed to processed supermarket bread), rye, wheat and other breads, can also be included. With a little detective work, you'll uncover the right amount and type of carbohydrates that work for you.

The Glycaemic Index: Myth or Reality?

Have you ever been told not to eat carrots because they're high glycaemic? How about white potatoes? One of the most popular nutrition strategies over the past few decades is to follow a low glycaemic diet. The glycaemic index (GI) is a relative ranking of how quickly carbohydrates are absorbed into the bloodstream. High GI foods rush in quickly, low GI foods are slow and steady, and moderate GI foods are somewhere in between. Choosing foods based on the GI index is a strategy used by medical and nutrition professionals to maintain healthy glucose levels in clients. Does the research back up these claims? Let's review, starting with weight loss.

A recent meta-analysis in the *Canadian Journal of Diabetes* investigating over 1,500 overweight and obese individuals following low GI diets found it did not lead to greater weight loss than higher GI diets over a six-month period.[15] Strike one.

What about low GI diets and heart disease risk? A recent Cochrane Review meta-analysis of 21 randomized control trials concluded there is currently no evidence regarding the effects of low GI diets on cardiovascular disease.[16] Strike two.

How about combating chronic inflammation? Another large meta-analysis of 28 randomized control trials found no significant effect of low GI diets on reducing pro-inflammatory cytokines, the key messengers of inflammation.[17] Strike three.

Researchers recently concluded, 'A low glycaemic response alone does not necessarily justify a health claim.' In short, following a low-glycaemic diet is a good heuristic, or simple rule, to steer you towards more whole foods, not a clear path to success. A better simple rule is to eat food with one ingredient: carrots, potatoes, beef, lentils, broccoli, etc.

In short ... eat real food.

In Summary

Turning the dial on how much, or little, carbohydrate you should eat takes a little time. If you are struggling with weight gain, high blood pressure or high blood glucose levels, emerging evidence confirms your 'carbohydrate tolerance' – the amount of carbohydrates right for your activity levels and goals – plays a major role in your ability to keep blood glucose levels on point and maintaining your ideal weight.[18] Ratcheting down your carb intake will help to improve all of these areas. Depending on how much weight you have to lose, or your degree of insulin resistance, you'll need to experiment with your total carb intake to determine the right amount for you. (I'll discuss monitoring progress and making adjustments in Chapter 8.)

If you're already lean and looking to maximize performance, ratcheting up your carb intake around exercise (and ratcheting it down on rest days or at other meals), can help you find the right balance between body composition and performance.

———

In the summer of 2003, Kelly Holmes had to figure out how to fuel her training to recover from injury. The combination of insufficient calorie intake, lack of sleep and her high training load created the perfect storm for overtraining and injury. It was a daunting task to tackle, let alone whilst preparing for the biggest competition of her life to that point – the 2004 Olympic Games. Regardless of whether you're an elite athlete aiming for a podium finish, or you're trying to achieve your own personal weight-loss or performance goals, it's difficult to face the obstacles head on and experiment to find the right combination to overcome them and battle through it. The ability to put a plan in place, to trust the process and to adjust as needed is paramount to success and what separates elite athletes from the rest. Kelly Holmes trusted the process and with dogged effort and determination went on to win two gold medals in Athens in the 800 and 1,500 metres, fulfilling a lifelong dream. It didn't happen overnight: it took consistency and dedication to stay with the problem long enough to find a solution. There are no quick fixes. Commit yourself to the process, like Holmes, and you'll uncover the path to long-term success.

CHAPTER 8

Turn the Dial on Fats

'A smooth sea never made a skilled sailor.'
— **Franklin D. Roosevelt**, US president

I n 2005, British tennis player Andy Murray turned pro and the very next year he won his first Association of Tennis Professionals (ATP) title. In 2008, he reached his first Grand Slam final, losing to Roger Federer in the US Open. Murray seemed on the brink of winning his first major championship. Fast forward four years and he had made it to three more major finals and four major semi-finals, but lost all seven to the 'Big 3' of Roger Federer, Rafael Nadal and Novak Djokovic. (Adding salt to his wounds, he watched a player whom he routinely defeated as a junior, Novak Djokovic, win five majors during that time.) Despite the repeated disappointment, Murray refused to relent and decided to tackle the roadblocks head on, re-assessing every aspect of his game: training, sleep, recovery, nutrition, and so on. .

It's incredibly difficult to put in the work, day in and day out, in order to extract the smallest margin (regardless, of whether you're a pro or just trying to achieve your personal best). It takes a certain mindset. It takes willingness to embrace the uncertainty, to experiment, observe and adjust as needed. It also takes patience. These are the skills required to navigate the choppy waters of complex problems.

Confusing Fats

Understanding dietary fats is confusing. Not surprisingly, a recent survey of consumers regarding the role of fats in a healthy diet found 64 per cent felt confused by the contradictory messaging from governments, experts, food companies and the media.[1] If you're a little confused, too, you're not alone. Over 90 per cent of respondents also expressed a negative association to the term fat: women tend to associate fat with weight gain and men with poor heart health. Rightly or wrongly, these are the subconscious messages that stick, and when you're busy in mid life, it's hard to rewrite these deeply ingrained narratives.

If you look at trends in dietary fat consumption in America – which follow closely those in the UK, Australia and parts of Europe – fat intake has decreased from 36.6 to 33.6 per cent of calorie intake since the early 1970s, yet weight gain and diabetes have absolutely skyrocketed over that time.[2] The general public were told to reduce fat intake to trim their waistlines, yet the opposite occurred (largely to do with the massive rise in consumption of ultra-processed foods).

Reducing your fat intake (without subsequent weight loss) also does little for your overall health. Large studies, such as the Women's Health Initiative, found no benefit from lowering fat intake from 36 per cent to 29 per cent on the risk of heart disease, diabetes and cancers. Conversely, the PREDIMED and OmniHeart trials found health benefits when *increasing* healthy fats above the previously suggested 35 per cent of total calories mark in the Dietary Guidelines for Americans (this upper limit was removed in 2015).[3]

The Right Kind of Fat

When it comes to fats, quality matters most for keeping you healthy in mid life and beyond. The biggest problem with fats is the intake of ultra-processed food (yep, we're going to beat that drum again!). Trans fats, which will show up on food labels as partially hydrogenated oils, are the most common ingredient in mass-produced cakes, biscuits (cookies) and pies, as well as in microwave popcorn and frozen pizza, fried chicken, doughnuts, French fries and ready-made meals.

Why are trans fats so bad? They cause an absolute hurricane of damage to your cardiovascular system, increasing low-density lipoprotein cholesterol (LDL-c) and triglyceride levels, lowering protective high-density lipoprotein cholesterol (HDL-c), ramping up inflammation and damaging the innermost layer of your arterial walls.[4] Basically, everything that could possibly go wrong with your heart health biomarkers, goes wrong when you eat trans fats. So, what fats should you eat? Let's review.

Dietary Fats for Health in Mid Life

There are three main categories of fats: saturated, monounsaturated (MUFAs, pronounced *moo-fahs*) and polyunsaturated fats (PUFAs, pronounced *poo-fahs*).

In Chapter 6, I discussed the fundamental importance of protein intake and why you need to *Set Your Protein*. The challenge people face when aiming to consume more protein is the false narrative around saturated fat and the potential harmful effects on your health. Pay attention here because this is a *really important point* to understand. The majority of people are choosing not to eat red meat, dairy and eggs for 'health reasons', yet the research shows that omitting these foods is likely to cause more health problems than it solves. Let's do a deep dive.

Saturated Fat (from Animal Protein) Is Not the Problem

Stop me if you've heard this phrase before, 'I'm no longer eating red meat for health reasons.' You could also insert dairy into this phrase, with the segue into fake news about how it's 'pro-inflammatory'. The argument for avoiding or significantly limiting animal protein is largely based on the notion that they contain too many saturated fats, but there's a lot of nuance to this topic that gets overlooked. Limiting animal protein can, in fact, lead to poorer food choices and poorer diet quality, where people end up consuming more calories from processed carbs and/or fats.

How did we get to a point where 'real food' with one ingredient – beef, milk, egg, and the like – are still a public enemy, yet the heavily processed new vegan burger at your local grocery store that has an ingredients (and syllables) list as long as your arm is touted as a 'healthy' alternative? I love plant-based foods – lentils, brown rice, broccoli, avocado and the rest – but I don't love the heavily processed variety. Let's go back to the start.

In the late 1970s, the US issued their first set of dietary guidelines with a central theme of reducing saturated fat content below 10 per cent of total calories, in an effort to help reduce the rising tide of heart attacks and stroke. This recommendation for saturated fat still holds strong today; however, rates of heart attack and stroke have been on the rise in recent years.[5] It's created a debate even among experts: one group concluding there is *no evidence* to support the notion that reducing your saturated fat intake has any beneficial effect on lowering your risk of heart attack and stroke, while another found a beneficial effect of lowering saturated fat on heart disease risk.[6] Who are you to believe? You're not alone in your confusion; even the government is unsure. As a result, the US Departments of Agriculture and Health and Human Services recently decided to re-examine the relationship between saturated fat consumption (types and amounts) and risk of cardiovascular disease in adults.[7] Ultimately, the challenge with any complex problem is the high degree of uncertainty and ambiguity. You don't just eat saturated fats, you eat beef and the myriad of micronutrients and phytonutrients it contains, and so on.[8] Let's explore the nuances in saturated fatty acid intake from meat and dairy, and how it may influence your health.

Red Meat and Dairy and Cholesterol

The primary reason why many doctors, dietitians and scientists may fear red meat or dairy consumption (or for that matter an excess of saturated-fat-rich coconut oil) is because it can raise harmful, LDL-c concentration, a key biomarker associated with heart disease risk.[9]

Your doctor is correct in that high LDL-c levels are problematic for your health, because LDL-c plays a causal role in the development of atherosclerosis and heart disease.[10] There is also a general relationship between lowering your LDL-c and reducing your risk of heart attack and stroke.[11] As many cardiologists would say, 'It's the LDL-c, stupid!' (Total cholesterol has fallen out of favour because it's not predictive of heart events: half the people who suffer heart attacks have low cholesterol, the other half have high cholesterol.) But look deeper and expert lipidologists (scientists who study lipids, like LDL-c) are quick to point out the weakness of relying so heavily on one biomarker.

The Mediterranean Example

Let's examine the nutrition. If you reduce your saturated fat intake, your LDL-c levels may decline, but the reduction in LDL-c is primarily seen in large LDL-c molecules. Why is this important? Reducing your saturated fat intake by reducing red meat, dairy or eggs, does not lower the more dangerous, small dense LDL-c particles in the vast majority of people.[12] There are more ripple effects. When you reduce your saturated fatty acid consumption, you also lower high-density lipoprotein cholesterol (HDL-c) levels, well recognized as having a protective effect against heart and stroke. Not good. Finally, it's well accepted that the Mediterranean diet is the default 'diet of choice' for most medical professionals, due to its heart-health benefits. However, a curious footnote here is that the benefits people achieve on a Mediterranean-style diet occur without any remarkable changes in LDL-c.[13]

Let's dive deeper into a few real-world examples. By the year 2050, do you know which country will have the longest living people in the world? Spain. The Spanish population consumes above the recommended saturated fat intake target of 10 per cent of total calorie intake, yet experience only 38.9 deaths per 100,000 from heart disease.[14] For comparison, in America, the rate is more than double at 79.2 deaths per 100,000. How is this possible? It is food quality that matters.

Eat 'Real' Food

The key nuance is that Americans spend over 50 per cent of household income on ultra-processed foods (including processed meats), compared to a paltry 20.3 per cent in Spain. The Spanish eat more 'real' food, including more 'real' meat, not the processed burgers and hot dogs so prevalent in America. But it's not just the Spanish, the French also consume saturated fats above the recommended 10 per cent threshold, yet also have one of the longest life expectancies in the world, as well as only 30.9 heart disease deaths per 100,000. If red meat were causing health problems, wouldn't you see it in these populations (and others) around the world with the highest consumption? The French spend only 14.2 per cent of household income on ultra-processed foods.

The biggest contributors to saturated fat intake in the US, as per the National Health and Nutrition Examination survey and analysis by the National Cancer Institute, are pizza, desserts (grain-based and dairy), bacon, hamburgers and sausages.[15] Furthermore, the latest scientific research summarized by saying that it is highly unlikely that the saturated fat content of meat is responsible for correlation to increased heart disease risk.[16] Maybe the new refrain from cardiologists should read, '*It's the processed food, stupid!*'

Saturated Fats from Dairy: Why They're Different

Saturated fatty acids from dairy are different to other foods because they are *structurally* different. An often-overlooked nuance in the understanding of saturated fatty acids (SFAs) is the presence or absence of 'methyl branches' on the saturated fats carbon chain.

Dark Chocolate – Healthy but High in Saturated Fats

Dark chocolate has been found to be highly beneficial for heart health, blood pressure and even blood insulin levels.[17] The health benefits of dark chocolate appear to come from the high polyphenol, antioxidants and flavonol content. Dark chocolate is actually a top-10 polyphenol-rich food, making it an absolute antioxidant powerhouse.[18] What's interesting is that dark chocolate exerts these beneficial effects despite containing 23g saturated fat per 100g/3.5oz bar of 70 per cent Lindt chocolate. Compare this to a 100g serving of steak, which has 1.9g saturated fat, and even half a bar of 70 per cent Lindt chocolate will net you 5- to 6-fold increased intake. If saturated fat is so bad, why aren't doctors sounding the alarm against dark chocolate? In fact, most believe it's a benefit to health (which it is!).

Why is this important? Branched-chain SFAs found in dairy have similar physiological and biochemical properties to unsaturated fats, the fats more widely accepted to be health-promoting.[19]

For example, multiple meta-analysis studies have recently revealed that milk and yogurt consumptions are inversely associated with CVD risk.[20] That's right, including dairy products in your diet has been linked to fewer heart attacks and stroke (not more). Once again, the idea of including minimally processed foods holds strong. Milk and yogurt are all group 1 NOVA foods – raw and minimally processed foods. They also consist of a complex matrix of proteins, fatty acids, minerals like calcium and magnesium, vitamins like K2, bioactive peptides and probiotics and phospholipids. (Moderate amounts of cheese, a group 3 NOVA food, in your diet have also been found to support health.)

How about dairy consumption in specific chronic conditions like diabetes? A study of over 65,000 people from multiple countries around the world uncovered that higher saturated fat levels from dairy – measured in the blood and tissues – were strongly associated with a lower risk of diabetes.[21] Furthermore, full-fat dairy was linked to better outcomes in Type 2 diabetics.

The take-home message is that red meat, dairy and eggs do not *cause* chronic disease. That said, if you prefer not to eat meat and dairy, or you want to follow a strict plant-based approach, that's fine, just don't do so because you believe them to be unhealthy. The new science doesn't back that claim.

Still not convinced? Countries like Canada have jumped to the forefront and The Canadian Heart and Stroke Foundation recently removed any specific limitations on saturated fat intake in their recommendations and, instead, state that the Canadian Dietary

Guidelines 'do not include a threshold or limit for saturated fat and instead focus on a healthy dietary pattern'.[22] (Mic drop.)

Other Types of Fat

What about MUFAs? While not essential to the body (your body can make them from other fats), monounsaturated fats are found in abundance in Mediterranean-style diets, widely considered to be one of the healthiest dietary patterns on earth. Olive oil is the predominant fat source in Mediterranean diets and it contains phenolic compounds, like oleic acid, that exert antioxidant and anti-inflammatory effects.[23] Adding more olive oil to your meals can help protect your heart by increasing HDL-c, decreasing triglycerides and reducing blood pressure.

Nuts are also a good source of MUFAs and great for improving your blood lipid biomarkers. Over 60 studies on the addition of nuts to your diet found daily servings help to reduce

What about Coconut Oil?

There is a difference between *virgin* coconut oil and regular coconut oils. The majority of coconut oils in confectioneries, cakes and snacks are highly processed and hydrogenated, which raise your LDL-c levels. Whereas, more gently prepared virgin coconut oil appears not to.[24] In fact, when compared with olive oil, virgin coconut oil has been shown to have similar positive effects in healthy dietary patterns in humans.[25]

LDL-c.[26] That said, by far the most popular source of MUFAs these days are avocadoes. Hipsters and the growing plant-based community have made 'avo on toast' a staple in most restaurants and cafés. (Just add a glass of soy milk to kick up the protein intake.) A randomized study of daily avocado consumption in overweight and obese individuals resulted in a significant drop in LDL-c levels and the small, dense, harmful LDL-c particles.[27] Of course, avocadoes don't just contain health-promoting MUFAs, they're also a great source of fibre, magnesium, vitamins B5 and B6, folate, vitamin C and potassium, to name just a few. This is what makes nutrition so challenging for scientists – you cannot control for all the variables. Inferences must be made. Wisdom and clinical insight is important.

PUFAs are the last category of fats in the diet and omega-3 and omega-6 fats are both examples of PUFAs, and are considered essential in your diet, although deficiency is rare. While omega-3 fats get the most attention in the media, it's actually the ratio of the two that matters most. Today, the modern, ultra-processed diet has skewed the ratio of omega-6 to omega-3 from 15:1 to 20:1 in the general population, which is in stark contrast to traditional hunter-gatherer populations around the world, who consume a ratio of between 4:1 and 1:1.[28] These pre-industrial societies are largely free from chronic lifestyle diseases, like heart disease and diabetes. Omega-6 fats are not 'bad', but because they're used so extensively in processed and packaged foods for taste and texture, they can become very problematic when over-consumed, as they're easily oxidized in the body, sparking inflammation that can derail health over time. For example, soybean oil is the highest source of omega-6 fats in the American diet, largely due to its extensive use in processed foods, and is a major reason why omega-6 fatty acids found in body-fat stores have increased three-fold in the last 50 years.[29] Reducing your ultra-processed food intake reduces the excess intake of omega-6 fats.

The Problem with Our Modern Diet

What foods provide the bulk of our MUFAs intake? The following is a recent breakdown of intake in the general population – the percentage given is the amount that food contributes to an individual's MUFAs intake:

- Grain-based desserts, such as cakes and biscuits (cookies) (8.9 per cent)
- Chicken, sausages and bacon (7.6 per cent)
- Nuts and seeds (5.5 per cent)
- Pizzas (5.4 per cent)
- Fried foods (4.9 per cent)
- Burgers (4.5 per cent)[30]

Not exactly an all-star list of foods (with the exception of nuts and seeds). If you can simply reduce your intake of these ultra-processed convenience foods and replace them with 'real food' sources of oleic acid from olive oil, avocadoes and nuts, you'll lay the foundation for better health in mid life.

Increasing your omega-3 intake, by eating cold-water fatty fish, like sardines, salmon and mackerel, etc, is important because it provides the extra-long chain omega-3 fats DHA and EPA, which exert beneficial effects on health. However, it's not enough just to increase your omega-3 intake, you need to reduce your omega-6 intake as well. Once again, that means cutting down on your ultra-processed food consumption.

Step 4 - Turn the Dial on Your Fat Intake

While the science of dietary fats is complex, how it plays out in your diet doesn't have to be. When it comes to saturated fat, focus on reducing processed foods to keep saturated fat intake in check and don't go crazy with butter or coconut oil (use them in moderation). The more overweight or obese you are, the lower your intake should be. Focus on the quality of your diet and the fats you eat, rather than one specific food or nutrient. Don't sweat the small stuff. (That said, there is a little more nuance when it comes to weight loss.)

Here Is Your Fat Intake Plan
Eat 0.7–1.4g/kg per day, which is:
- Women – 1–2 'thumbs' per meal
- Men – 2–3 'thumbs' per meal

When to Eat
Timing is not very important.
Divide intake evenly throughout meals of the day.

Fat Type - Choose From
Saturated fats
- From animal protein
- Modest amounts of butter or virgin coconut oil, when cooking or added to food

MUFAs
- Olives
- Olive oil (extra-virgin)
- Avocadoes
- Rapeseed/Canola oil
- Nuts: almonds, cashews, macadamias, pecans, walnuts, etc

PUFAs
- Omega-3 – Primary:
  - Fish: salmon, mackerel, anchovies, sardines, herring, black cod, etc
  - Seafood: mussels, scallops, oysters, clams, etc
- Omega-3 – Secondary:
  - Eggs
  - Grass-fed beef
  - Sea algae

What to Cook With

Low-moderate heat – olive oil (extra-virgin) or rapeseed/canola oil

High heat – butter, ghee, beef tallow or duck fat

Note: most cooking should be done at low-moderate heat to support health.

Adjusting Fat (and Carb)
Intake to Lose Weight

Let's look into the future.... You've adjusted your food intake and the majority of your diet is made up of healthy fats from real food. Your energy is better, your health is improving, but there is one small snag – you're still not losing weight. This is when you can get 'too much of a good thing'. When it comes to losing weight, you should turn the dial down on either carbohydrates or fats. How much do you need to drop energy intake to trigger fat loss? A reduction between 300–500 calories per day (from carbohydrates or fats, or a combination of both), throughout the week, should be sufficient to trigger fat loss.

If getting leaner is your goal, at some point you'll need to trim dietary fat intake to continue to make progress. Fats contain 9 calories per gram, compared to only 4 calories per gram for carbohydrates, which means energy intake drops quickly when you reduce your fat intake. For example, switching from full-fat Greek yogurt to a low-fat, low-sugar version, reducing your intake of nuts, nut butters, spreads like hummus, or the amount of oils you cook with, are all possible strategies to trim your daily calorie intake.

Does This Mean a Low-Fat Diet?

Not at all. It simply means you're going to apply a targeted strategy to achieve a desired outcome. The strategy that works best for you may be different from your friend, family member or colleague at work (this is where personalization comes into play). You may include a certain amount of low-fat meals per day or a certain amount of lower fat days per week. It's not a 'one size fits all' approach.

Assessing Progress

The key with weight loss is that you want to lose weight as gradually as possible by eating as much as possible (not as little). Physiologically, you can only lose about 0.5–1.0 per cent of your body weight per week from fat. Any additional weight that comes off is from muscle (not good), glycogen stores (also not good) and water (really not good). Starve yourself and this is precisely what you'll be losing; not a strategy for long-term success. Rapid weight loss might feel great in month one, but it will inevitably lead to stalled progress in month two or three, and then reverting back to where you started by month three or four.

How can you track progress?

If you weigh yourself 2–3 times per week, you can take a 'weekly average' of those measurements. Using the weekly average, you can then gauge your progress.

Did you lose at least 0.5 per cent of your body weight last week?

If yes, continue with your nutrition and exercise plan. If not, you'll need to reduce dietary intake by another 300–500 calories per day (or increase energy expenditure via exercise; more on this in Section Three).

Getting more granular with your assessment will help highlight the effects of your dietary and exercise changes. You'll learn how much (or little) you need to *Turn the Dials* on carb and fat intakes to achieve your goals. But, once again, it doesn't mean you're signing yourself up for a lifetime of tracking. It's simply an exercise to build the skills required to succeed in the long run.

Blood Test Biomarkers to Track Health Progress

Blood test biomarkers from your annual physical check-up can provide a wealth of information on the impact that your diet, exercise and lifestyle changes are having on your health. The following is a run-down of biomarkers to track.

Fasting Glucose

Fasting glucose levels measured first thing in the morning provide you with a snapshot of your overall health. Aim to achieve consistent readings below 94mg/dL (5.2mmol/L), as this has been associated with the lowest levels of mortality from any cause, regardless of sex or age.[31] Remember, it's not just your diet that impacts fasting glucose; insufficient sleep, chronic stress and overtraining can all raise your fasting glucose measure.

HbA1c

Haemoglobin A1c is a blood test that provides a snapshot of your estimated three-month average of blood glucose level. It's a great baseline to assess general health. Aim for levels at 5.4 per cent or lower. Remember, HbA1c has a time dependency, which means it reflects your more recent levels of blood glucose.[32]

Tg/HDL Ratio

The ratio of your triglycerides to your HDL-c levels (Tg/HDL) is a cheap and cheerful proxy for assessing your insulin sensitivity (otherwise only measurable in a research lab setting) and a strong predictor of healthy ageing in mid life and beyond.[33] The optimal range is between 0.5–1.9, whereas some insulin resistance is likely from 2.0–3.0 and, if you score above 3.0, you're at significant risk of insulin resistance and heart disease.

Apo B:Apo A1 Ratio

A much closer approximation of your heart attack and stroke risk is the ratio of apolipoprotein B (apo B) found on every LDL-c molecule and apolipoprotein A1 (apo A1) found on every HDL-c molecule. Thus, the ApoB:ApoA1 ratio represents the balance between heart disease 'causing' and 'preventing' lipoproteins. New research continues to support the strong association between ApoB:ApoA1 ratio and the severity of heart disease, as well as potentially being a better predictor of clinical outcomes.[34] The prestigious Mayo Clinic reports that if your ApoB:ApoA1 ratio is less than 0.7 for men and 0.6 for women, you're at low risk; between 0.7–0.9 for men and 0.6–0.8 for women, you're at average risk; and greater than 0.9 for men and 0.8 for women, you're at high risk of heart disease and mortality.

Interestingly, eating avocado daily improves your ApoB:ApoA1 ratio.[35]

GGT (Liver Enzyme)
GGT is a liver enzyme associated with blood sugar dysfunction, insulin resistance and fatty liver disease. It's one of the earliest red flags for poor metabolic health. The desired range for GGT is less than 30 U/L.

hs-CRP
CRP (C-reactive protein) is a measure of overall systemic inflammation. Typically, the more overweight or out of shape you are, the greater your inflammatory levels. The desired range is less than 1.0mg/L.

After the 2011 season, Andy Murray reassessed his game and worked tirelessly in the off-season to close the gap on the 'Big 3'. In 2012, his hard work and consistent effort paid off. Murray became the first male British player to reach the finals at Wimbledon. Sadly, he lost to Federer in the final. Undeterred, he played Federer again just a few weeks later in the 2012 London Olympic Games final at the exact same venue; this time, beating Federer in straight sets to win an Olympic gold medal. Less than two months after that, Murray went on to win his first major championship at the US Open, defeating Djokovic in a five-set thriller. Complex problems take time to solve, but the journey (and effort required) makes the taste of victory that much sweeter.

SECTION THREE

Rebuild and Recover

CHAPTER 9

Leaner, Faster, Stronger

'Exercise is king.'

—JACK LALANNE, fitness and nutrition expert

Jonny Wilkinson is one of the great all-time English rugby players, but he could have been *the* greatest. He was a crucial member of the team during one of England's most dominant periods in rugby in the early 2000s. During that span, they defeated every other nation in the world, including stalwarts New Zealand and Australia. They won three Six Nations titles and went on to glory by winning the 2003 World Cup Final in Sydney, Australia. After Wilkinson's incredible performance in that final, his career was derailed by multiple injuries. A torn knee ligament and arm and shoulder problems left Wilkinson sidelined for the better part of three years. It would've been easy for him to retire and be content with his 'glory years'. But his own goals and passion for the game pushed him to keep rehabbing, keep training and keep showing up every day, in order to achieve his dream – to play in another World Cup.

What's Holding You Back?

The challenge in mid life is that exercise is not the same as when you were younger. This is true whether you're an elite athlete or simply trying to keep fit. The warm-up takes longer (much longer!) and you need to be more cautious with your lifts or how many miles you log. You also struggle simply to carve out half an hour to exercise (and this feels like an achievement!). If you do get outside for that morning run, your knee starts acting up after the endorphins wear off. And if you get back into the gym, your lower back starts stiffening up later in the day, after the adrenaline subsides.

To pursue your passions and fulfil your PEAK40 goals, you need to be resilient, both mentally and physically. The act of building physical strength will assist in creating mental strength, but, to achieve success, you must be consistent with your efforts and, in order to do so, you've got to stop the pain train. Like Wilkinson, you need to rebuild your body. All those hours slumped over your desk, sitting in your car, or slouched on the sofa, and the nights sitting up awkwardly with your kids, have led to what feels like a broken you. You may have noticed that when you feel physically weak, stiff or in pain, your mental state tends to follow suit. Is this your destiny in mid life and beyond? Not at all.

It doesn't matter if you've never played a sport in your life or whether you were an all-star athlete, movement is hard-wired into your DNA over millions of years of evolution – you were born to move. It's time to reconnect with your inner athlete, even though it feels like another item on your to-do list. Exercise is a powerful tool for igniting better health, lifting your mood, building muscle and shedding body fat – especially in mid life. Let's explore.

Movement Is Medicine

It is an unfortunate fact that the more weight you gain, the more likely you are to struggle with heart disease, Type 2 diabetes, cancer and other chronic conditions.[1] Specifically, high belly fat is independently associated with death by any cause and is actually a better predictor of obesity-related conditions than either body weight or BMI.[2] Diet plays a major role in weight gain and poor health, but so too does inactivity.

Physical inactivity is strongly associated with all chronic disease conditions.[3] Movement is a primary means of prevention as it reduces your risk of obesity, cardiovascular disease, diabetes, cancer, respiratory disorders and the like.[4] The power of exercise is so robust that even if you're diagnosed with a chronic condition, adding exercise to your medical treatment plan improves your quality of life.[5]

Bulletproof Your Health in Mid Life

No drug in the world can do what movement can for your health.[6] Virtually every physiological system is affected by exercise. Movement:

- improves the strength of your heart muscles and their ability to deliver oxygen
- lowers blood pressure, reduces inflammation and stress hormone levels
- increases protective HDL-c (e.g. ApoA1)
- and enhances weight loss

If you move daily, you reduce your risk of heart attack and stroke by 80 per cent, Type 2 diabetes by 90 per cent and cancer by 33 per cent.

Movement also upgrades your mental performance. Regular physical activity improves the structure and functions of the neurons in your brain, ramping up learning and skill acquisition (even if you're already a healthy adult).

With all these benefits, you would think exercise was a lifestyle staple for everyone in mid life, but alarmingly only 15–20 per cent of people achieve the recommended guidelines of 150 minutes of moderate-intense activity per week, or at least 75 minutes of vigorous activity.[7] By mid life, 33 per cent of adults fail to engage in any type of physical activity.[8]

So, why don't people get enough exercise? One big challenge is that movement has been reverse-engineered out of our lives. Why take the stairs at work when the elevator is right there (can you even find the stairs in your building?)? Why cook a homemade meal when companies will deliver with no effort? Why go out for a walk to meet up with friends when you can chat on social media?

Of course, in mid life it's also the sheer volume of life demands that extinguishes free time. Your increasingly congested schedule doesn't *seem* to allow time for exercise. The keyword here is seem – time management is really priority management. When you begin to prioritize movement over other things, small opportunities for more movement will reveal themselves in your day. There *is* time for more movement in your life; the opportunities are all around you.

From Stiff Penguin to Supple Leopard

In his ground-breaking book *Becoming A Supple Leopard*, Kelly Starrett, PhD, physiotherapist and movement specialist to the pros, created the 'how to' bible for getting yourself unstuck and moving freely again. Starrett highlighted that pain, swelling, numbness, tingling and the like are all latent indicators of deeper problems that have been developing for some time. He also points out that movement will override pain, which was protective from an evolutionary standpoint for survival but creates problems in the present because you don't realize you're in pain until you lie down and feel your back or shoulder throbbing.

Finally, Starrett spotlights our societal obsession with 'completing tasks', like finishing the marathon or deadlifting a personal best, at the expense of plantar fasciitis or a herniated disc.

Rather than prioritizing your ability to complete the task, take a moment to observe the quality of your movement or positioning. Do your knees stick up towards the ceiling when you sit cross-legged? Are you able to touch your toes? Can you scratch the middle of your back? Tensions in all of these key areas – hips, lower and upper back, and shoulders – make it difficult to jump right into an exercise programme. One of the biggest challenges in modern life is that it rarely puts your body through a full range of motion and, over time, your body will stiffen and grow tense. Even if you're athletic and not aware of any irregular movement tendencies, years of weight-lifting can leave you stuck in the same predicament.

To get moving easily again and reach PEAK40 fitness, you need to be pain free. This means addressing your lack of mobility. A simple place to start is to do some 1950s style calisthenics: simply moving your joints around from your ankles all the way up to your shoulders, neck and head. Disciplines like tai chi or yoga are also very beneficial for restoring movement.

Build Your Aerobic Base (and Be Efficient)

Common questions I get asked by clients are, 'What's the best exercise to improve my health?' or 'What's the best exercise to lose weight?' The challenge for researchers when trying to uncover the 'best' type of any exercise is the fact that it depends on the individual's goals. The aim in mid life is to achieve strength and fitness in the most efficient manner possible and the good news is *both* resistance training (i.e. lifting weights or heavy objects) and aerobic training (i.e. cardiovascular conditioning) can reduce body mass index (BMI), blood pressure and improve aerobic fitness.[9]

Stretches to Do at Home

Try these three movements/positions:

Crossed-Legged Work Station

Sit crossed-legged on the floor or carpet whilst doing laptop work or watching TV, rather than sitting on a chair or couch. Work in this position for 5–10 minutes, building up your ability to tolerate it. This will help to improve hip mobility.

The Lunging Laptop

Use the corner of your bed or couch as a table. Get into a lunge position, with one leg extended behind you. Work in this position for 5–10 minutes, building up your ability to tolerate it. This will stretch your psoas muscle, the deep hip flexor that extends into your lower back.

Superman Hold

Take a break from work or do this at the end of a day. Lie face down on the carpet, keeping your lower body firmly on the ground. Squeeze your glutes and lift your upper body, holding your arms out at your side (thumbs pointing towards the ceiling). Hold for 5–10 seconds and repeat 2–5 times.

There are countless strategies to incorporate more mobility into your day. Go to DrBubbs.com/PEAK40 to check out free videos on how to get started.

Upgrade Your Aerobic Fitness

Let's start by exploring the benefits of aerobic fitness on health, weight loss and longevity. If you're not a runner by nature, fear not, you don't need to commit to training for a marathon (unless you want to!), you simply need to upgrade your aerobic base. Aerobic fitness is a powerful tool in mid life for improving your heart health, blood glucose control and insulin sensitivity, as well as regulating appetite hormones, reducing belly fat and giving you a mental boost.[10] It is also strongly linked to longevity and healthy ageing. And you can start with something as simple as walking.

Walking is a very under-appreciated form of physical activity. A recent study of sedentary, overweight, mid-life men and women aged 35–59 years with mildly elevated blood pressure and blood glucose levels revealed some compelling results. Participants were asked to increase their steps per day from 4,000 to a *minimum* of 10,000 steps per day to see what effect this 2.5-fold increase would have on their blood pressure. After completing the 12-week programme, the group logging 10k steps daily experienced a 13.7mmHg drop in blood pressure and a 14.9mg/dL (0.8mmol/L) drop in fasting blood glucose.[11] Incredible to think something as simple as walking could yield results on par (or better) than medications.

Cycling is another great option to build aerobic fitness with low impact on the joints. In 2020, at the annual meeting of the European Association for the Study of Diabetes, researchers from Denmark found that cycling for only 1 hour per week was linked to a 25 per cent decrease in death by any cause, compared to those who didn't cycle.[12] When participants bumped up their cycling to at least 2.5 hours per week, they experienced a 31 per cent drop. That's an astounding benefit when you think that 2.5 hours per week is the equivalent of cycling for just over 20 minutes a day.

Time-Efficient Aerobic Exercise

In light of the fact that most people don't achieve the recommended weekly dose of exercise, often because they can't find enough time, scientists have been exploring more time-efficient modes of exercise, or combinations of types of exercise, to shrink the time-commitment gap that prevents most people from even getting started. How can you be more time-efficient with your exercise? Dr Martin Gibala, PhD, from McMaster University in Canada, has been studying high-intensity interval training (HIIT) and its many variations for decades. Gibala's work was pivotal in the field – it was the first to show that 1 minute of exercise (3 × 20 second bursts) done three times per week could elicit the same benefit as the government-recommended 150 minutes weekly.[13] His work has also uncovered time-efficient HIIT strategies that can help lower blood pressure, blood glucose levels, and inflammation and improve endothelial function (the innermost lining of your arteries). It's especially potent for reversing Type 2 diabetes – in 2020, researchers in Taiwan found people with Type 2 diabetes reduced their risk of death (by any cause) by a whopping 25–32 per cent with high intensity exercise.[14]

In his terrific book, *The One Minute Workout*, Gibala outlines his research on HIIT training for health and weight loss, and shares simple strategies for HIIT workouts that are 30 minutes or less. The two sessions that I've found work really well are the Wingate Classic and the 10 × 1 (see 'Step 1' on pages 121–123).

What about Steady-State Cardio?

Does that mean steady-state cardio (your typical jog or cycle at a conversational pace) isn't helpful? Not so fast. Referred to as moderate intensity continuous training (MICT) in the research, steady-state cardio is actually *more* impactful for improving long-term glucose control than HIIT.[15]

The Power of Coffee

Coffee is a powerful weapon for improving fitness, body composition and longevity. Coffee contains a complex mixture of over 1,000 bioactive compounds – including caffeine, chlorogenic acids and cafestol – which exert potent antioxidant, anti-inflammatory and anti-ageing benefits.[16] A coffee before your morning exercise (caffeine is also found in black and green tea in lower doses) helps to ignite your morning workout by increasing alertness and 'feel good' endorphin release, as well as reducing the perceived exertion of training (i.e. exercise feels easier).[17]

Caffeine also helps to promote the breakdown of body fat for fuel during exercise. The benefits don't stop there. When it comes to longevity, a recent large meta-analysis concluded that regular coffee consumption was associated with lower risk of cardiovascular mortality, cancer and death by any cause.[18] Impressive benefits, to say the least. The 'sweet spot', in order to maximize the benefits of caffeine and limit adverse symptoms (i.e. irritability, restlessness, anxiety and insomnia), appears to be 2–3mg caffeine per kilogram of your body weight per day. For most people, this is the equivalent of 1–2 coffees per day.

Steady-state cardio is also great for reducing belly fat. Compared head-to-head with resistance training, a recent, large analysis of 43 studies found aerobic exercise reduced belly fat the most (although resistance training did reduce belly fat, too, just not as much).[19] The benefit isn't just aesthetic. Reduction in belly fat is associated with a reduction in death by any cause and is now recognized as a better predictor of obesity-related conditions than either increased body weight or BMI.[20]

Bulletproof Your Body: Build Muscle

Stress of any kind is essential for growth, whether of muscle, bone or brain. Stress provides the 'signal' to become stronger, faster and leaner. Resistance training, like lifting weights or using resistance bands, provides the stress from which your muscles, ligaments and bones grow stronger. We've evolved to bend, squat, lift and carry heavy things. The more you incorporate these into your daily life, the better your health and the easier it is to maintain a healthy body composition.

If you're new to training, the early adaptations are primarily due to your nervous system becoming more efficient at sending the signals to your muscles to tell them to contract, referred to by muscle scientists as muscular activation.[21] Building muscle mass (or maintaining what you already have), is largely driven by three main factors: mechanical tension, metabolic stress and muscle damage. Mechanical tension is the stress imposed on your muscles by a load like a barbell or dumbbell. Metabolic stress is the build up of metabolites, like lactate, in your muscle cells during exercise. Lastly, muscle damage is the physical damage to the muscle cell due to exercise.

In mid life, the goal is to be efficient with your training because you don't have a lot of time to exercise. So, what factor contributes most to muscle building? Expert muscle scientist Dr Brad Schoenfeld, PhD, says the evidence points to mechanical tension.[22] Special receptors in your muscles sense how heavy, and for how long, you lift a barbell, dumbbell or heavy bag of

Step 1 - Restore Your Aerobic Fitness

Higher intensity (HIIT) workouts and sprinting are best for upgrading your heart health and fitness.

Steady-state cardio is great for building an aerobic base, improving glucose control and trimming belly fat.

Two HIIT Workouts

The Wingate Classic. After a 3–5-minute warm-up on a stationary bicycle, push yourself very hard for 30 seconds, (i.e. reaching an 8 or 9 of perceived exertion on a scale of 1–10), followed by a 4.5-minute rest. (If you do it right and push yourself hard enough, you'll need every second of rest!) Complete five rounds and then cool down.

10 × 1. After a 3–5-minute warm-up on a stationary bicycle, perform 1 moderate-to-hard minute (at an intensity of approximately 7 on a scale of 1–10), followed by a 1-minute rest (which will go by in the blink of an eye). On the next round, push the intensity a little higher during the 'work' interval. Repeat for 5–6 intervals in your first week, then cool down. Add an extra round every week until you reach a total of 10 intervals.

Sprint to Better Health and Body Composition
Sprinting is phenomenal for your health, but you have to build up to it gradually. In my first book,

Peak: The New Science of Athletic Performance That Is Revolutionizing Sports, I share the work of Jason Hettler, lead strength and speed development coach at ALTIS in Arizona, an elite track and field training facility and home to the 'best of the best' track and field athletes in the world.

Hettler works with world-class sprinters and consults with professional sports teams on how to develop better sprinting qualities in team sport athletes. But the benefits can extend beyond the professionals. If you're looking to improve aerobic fitness, speed and mobility (and even get leaner as well!), it can help. You used to sprint naturally as a kid but over the years, you may have gradually stopped. If your body is injury free and you're feeling fitter, it's time to rediscover the joy of sprinting. Where do you start if you want to add sprinting into your regime? Here are a few tips from coach Hettler:

- Be patient. It takes time to build sprinting 'skills'.
- Use the warm-up to improve your mobility and learn the skills.
- Start off on grass, rather than a track or hard surface (to reduce ground-force impact).
- Build acceleration with sprints from 20–30 metres (elite sprinters accelerate for up to 50m!).
- Build speed at distances of 30–60 metres (elite sprinters do this over 50–90 metres).

- Build speed endurance at 60 metres+ (elite sprinters do this at 90 metres+).
- To help get your rhythm, skip into the start of your sprint, referred to as a 'drop-in'. This can reduce the force of overcoming the inertia of starting from a standstill. If you're a novice, Hettler suggests using drop-ins to reduce the impact and stress on your body. Over time and as your form improves, you'll adapt to the physical demands. Like any skill, the results are amplified with regular practice.

Build Your Aerobic Base with Steady-State Training

- First, make sure your ankles, knees, hips and lower back are in good health.
- Find a distance or type of training you like, and remember to start small so you can be consistent with effort over the year.
- Build up your mileage gradually over time. Aim for 3–5 days of running or walk-running per week (this can include HIIT sessions).

Don't forget these aerobic sessions are great 'recovery runs', improving blood flow and accelerating recovery from strenuous HIIT exercise (and the rest of your gruelling work day). (Go to DrBubbs.com/PEAK40 to download your full base-building cardio plan.)

groceries for that matter, which then provides the greatest stimulus to build muscle.

Go Lighter If You Need to

But what if you've experienced quite a few injuries in your life or struggle with joint or lower back pain? Should you lift heavy loads? In mid life, tension has built up over the years in muscles and joints, so it's great to know the research shows you can achieve positive gains in muscle mass with lighter loads, so long as you train to failure (i.e. until you cannot complete another repetition with good form).[23] Research in older adults shows that you can train at 40 per cent of your 1-repetition maximum and still reap almost all the benefits of using weights, if you train to failure. You do have to push yourself, but even if you don't have access to a gym or weights, you can still make significant gains.

Lastly, muscle damage is probably the most misunderstood element of building muscle. You often read about the importance of damaging muscle tissue with intense workouts, however, this angle is over-hyped. The research clearly shows you don't want to damage your muscles too significantly, because excessive damage limits adaptation and holds you back from maximizing muscle growth. You shouldn't be sore for more than two days after a workout; if you are, you've likely pushed a little too hard. Just do enough to elicit a stress on the muscles, then, in the next session, do a little more.

Minimum-Effective Dose for Strength Training

Research shows resistance training can improve your metabolic health and protect against pre-diabetes and diabetes, lower chronic inflammation and improve your HbA1c levels (three-month average of blood glucose).[24] What's the ideal dose of resistance exercise in mid life?

Step 2 - Rebuild Your Strength

Aiming for the minimum effective dose helps to minimize the wear and tear on your joints and maximize your muscle-building benefits. Dr Brad Schoenfeld, PhD, found that the minimum effective dose is 10 sets per body part, per week.[25] That's all.

What Does This Look Like in Practice?

- 5 sets of squats for approximately 10–20 repetitions, followed by 5 sets of a 'push' exercise, like a dumbbell (DB) bench press, and 5 sets of a 'pull' upper-body exercise, like a seated row.
- On another day, 5 sets of deadlifts, followed by 5 sets of a 'push' exercise, like an overhead press, and 5 sets of a 'pull' upper body exercise, like a lat pulldown or chin-up.

Of course, you can add 1–2 sets of 'accessory' exercises for smaller muscle groups, like arms, shoulders, calves and core, at the end of your workout and it will still only take you about 25–30 minutes to complete the session (see Table 9.1 for a list of exercises).

Remember, strength training isn't just about your muscles, it's about restoring natural movement patterns for pain-free living, better energy and overall health.

Go to DrBubbs.com/PEAK40 to check out free videos on technique, form and how to get started.

Table 9.1. Exercise Selection for Minimum-Effective-Dose Training

Exercise - Day 1	Sets	Reps	Rest
A1) Squats	5	10	—
A2) DB Chest Press	5	12	60s
B1) Accessory Lifts (select from list I)	3	15	—
B2) Accessory Lifts (select from list II)	3	15	60s
C1) Core – Hollow Rock	2	10–20	60s
Exercise - Day 2	**Sets**	**Reps**	**Rest**
A1) Deadlift	5	10	—
A2) Push-Ups (45-degree incline)	5	10–16	60s
B1) Accessory Lifts (select from list I)	3	20	—
B2) Accessory Lifts (select from list II)	3	20	60s
C1) Core – Side Plank (each side)	2	20–40	60s

Accessory Lifts

List I

Cable Row – Rope (Elbow Out)

Face Pull – Rope

DB Row – Single-Arm (Elbow Out)

DB Pullover

List II

DB Seated External Rotation

DB Scarecrows

DB Lateral Raise + External Rotation

Band Pull Apart

The Benefits of Body-Weight Training

Don't have any weights at home? Or maybe you have a history of injury? No problem. If you train with body-weight exercises, such as squats and push-ups, it's not just the mechanical tension contributing to the effect, metabolic stress also plays an important role. You've probably experienced it when performing a circuit-type training – it's the 'burn' that builds up in your muscles from the accumulation of lactic acid and hydrogen ions. You can increase the metabolic effect of your work-out by reducing rest periods, allowing for only 30 seconds of rest, for example, rather than 60 seconds.

Boost Your Mood

Pumping iron is a powerful tool for boosting mood. *The Journal of the American Medical Association Psychiatry* recently analyzed 33 clinical trials to investigate the effects of resistance exercise on depression and found it 'significantly reduced depressive symptoms' among participants.[26] Lifting heavy things is built into our DNA as humans and you don't necessarily need to hit the gym to get started – carry a heavy bag of groceries home; perform walking lunges in the park; or use the bench to do step-ups. There are opportunities to exercise all around you.

Strengthen Your Immunity

If you're looking to improve your immune function, exercise is a fundamental piece of the puzzle. The fitter you are, the lower your likelihood of infection. Exercise strengthens your immune system, so it's better equipped to deal with the next round of infections.[27] Research shows that if you do get sick, exercise helps to reduce the severity and duration of your illness. There has perhaps never been a better time to start exercising.

Be Realistic So You Can Be Consistent

The best predictor for achieving your exercise goals is consistency, regardless of whether it's aerobic or resistance training. Concurrent training is when you perform resistance and aerobic training at the same time, which will yield the best results for you in mid life. That said, many ex-athletes still fear the 'interference effect' – the phenomenon of how aerobic training can reduce the gains you make when lifting weights (interestingly, this effect does not occur in the reverse direction; strength training has no adverse effect on endurance performance and can actually improve it). Unless you're competing as a powerlifter or bodybuilder, you don't need to worry about the interference effect. Even elite rugby players, a sport with heavy power, strength and aerobic demands, are not hindered by the interference effect. But a good rule of thumb, if you are worried, is to perform strength training and cardio on separate days. Lastly, be realistic about your expectations. Adding half a kilo or one pound of muscle in a month is tremendous progress, although it won't seem like much. You need to be consistent over months (and years!) to achieve significant goals. Building the right habits is key to achieving compliance and consistency; motivation and discipline won't get you all the way home, the road is simply too long. Most people are way too ambitious in January (or when starting a new programme) when inspiration and motivation are high, but when the spark fizzles out, so too does compliance. Exercise is about consistency. If you show up every week, all year, you'll be rewarded.

Leaner, Faster, Stronger: Training Plan Summary

Incorporate 1–2 HIIT sessions per week, along with steady-state cardio as a 'recovery' tool to build aerobic fitness, which is strongly linked to healthy ageing and longevity.

For resistance training, two days of lifting per week is your minimum effective dose, increasing to three days if your schedule permits. (Go to DrBubbs.com /PEAK40 to download the 30-day programme.)

Remember, you need to make time for exercise. You need to prioritize physical activity and schedule it into your day as if your mental and physical health depend on it, because in many ways, they do.

Remember, you'll never achieve your PEAK40 goals if you're in constant pain and discomfort. World-class athletes like Jonny Wilkinson know this all too well. In his first game back after more than three years of battling chronic pain and injury, Wilkinson set a record, scoring 27 points in the Calcutta Cup, earning him Man of the Match. The following week, he became the highest point scorer in the history of the Six Nations Championship. Then, Wilkinson fulfilled his ultimate goal, after battling back from all those injuries, he played a pivotal role in England's run to the 2007 World Cup Final. The opening game of that tournament was 1,169 days after his last appearance for England. His positive attitude and consistent daily efforts over that time span – in the clinic rehabbing, in the weights room and on the pitch – led to his exceptional results. Your attitude, effort and consistency will lead to exceptional results in your life as well.

CHAPTER 10

Recovery Starts with Sleep

'I'll sleep when I'm dead.'
— WARREN ZEVON, musician

I t's 2010. World-class British marathon runner Paula Radcliffe wakes up around 7.30am and takes her resting heart rate while her young daughter Isla sleeps. Radcliffe is the fastest female marathon runner of all time and a three-time winner of both the London and New York Marathons. Her resting heart rate is usually between 38–40 beats per minute (bpm), but when she starts training hard it climbs a little bit to about 42 bpm. This increase in resting heart rate is a physiological response to her higher training load, highlighting that her body is under stress. If she plans her training and recovery appropriately, it will allow her to peak for competition. If not, she'll overtrain and fail to keep up with the competition. It's a fine line in elite endurance sport. You must push your body to the edge, but not go over it. (Surviving the daily grind in mid life can feel quite similar!) If Paula's resting heart rate gets over 45 bpm, she knows she's pushing the needle too far into the red zone and she'll need to adjust her training plan to ensure proper recovery. Elite coaches will tell you that Olympic and pro athletes can push themselves hard and, more often than not, coaches need to pull them back. Where do they start with recovery? Sleep. Radcliffe would typically sleep from 10.30pm to 7.30am: a total of 9 hours' sleep. Lack of sleep impacts an athlete's speed, agility and ability to push through pain, it increases injury risk and reduces mental performance, immunity and the ability to recover. It can be the difference between winning and losing. If you're trying to upgrade your performance at work and home, sleep makes all the difference in the world to your ability to keep up with life's demands.

Start with Sleep

Lack of sleep destroys mental and physical health. There is almost nothing that can derail your health faster than insufficient sleep. Lack of sleep is strongly associated with:

- increased risk of Type 2 diabetes
- cardiovascular disease
- cancer
- dementia
- depression and anxiety
- mortality[1]

Lack of sleep also:

- pummels your immune system, increasing your susceptibility to cold and flu
- worsens your blood sugar control, causing a constant rollercoaster of energy highs and lows throughout the day
- increases your daily calorie intake by an average of just over 200 calories per day (might not sound like much, by it adds up in the long run)
- lowers testosterone levels by 10–20 per cent and zaps your libido[2]

On a day-to-day basis, lack of sleep wreaks havoc on your mental health, too, impairing your cognition, decision-making and ability to problem-solve and consolidate memories. It is while you are asleep that your brain performs critical housekeeping tasks: clearing out unnecessary clutter and toxins that build throughout the day; rebuilding the body via signalling your cells to repair any damaged DNA; and synergizing all the information we've taken in that day. As you accumulate a growing sleep debt, it worsens subjective measures of well-being, like fatigue, mood, muscle soreness, depression and confusion. If you're struggling with low mood or anxiety, lack of sleep contributes in a major way.

That's not all, the pitfalls continue. Insufficient sleep also makes you more likely to experience pain and reduces your ability to tolerate pain by approximately 10 per cent.[3] Insufficient sleep also leaves you more prone to injury.

If you're active and feeling pretty good, you're still not immune to the adverse effects of insufficient sleep. If you fail to achieve 8 hours' sleep per night, you're at 1.7 times greater risk of injury, compared to those who get at least 8 hours.[4] If you're an exercise enthusiast who likes to compete on the weekends, cumulative lack of weekday sleep negatively affects your performance on the weekend through poorer reaction times.[5]

There's a reason Paula Radcliffe aims for 8–9 hours' sleep; it enhances her recovery and thus propels her performance. But in mid life, life becomes so busy, sleep gets the short end of the stick. If you need more hours for work, family and friends or training, you typically have to sacrifice sleep to make it happen. Not only that, by mid life you've accumulated a large sleep debt (as you likely already know). If you've got kids, you may be getting woken up periodically through the night. So, what do you do now? Unfortunately, there are no short-cuts; the need for sleep has not changed in more than two million years of evolution. But you can get strategic with how you improve sleep quality and nudge forward your total sleep time to enhance all areas of mental and physical health.

How Much Sleep?

The National Sleep Foundation recommends adults get 7–9 hours' sleep per night.[6] However, almost two-thirds of adults worldwide report not getting enough sleep.[7] The typical person only gets about 6.5 hours per night and almost 50 per cent of Americans admit to suffering health consequences as a result. Alarmingly, 30 per cent of the population get less than 6 hours' sleep per night, further exacerbating these risks. If you consider that even one night of poor sleep increases rates of workplace injury and heart attacks, and seven days of less than 6 hours leaves your mental state equivalent to a person legally intoxicated, what does half a decade or more of poor or interrupted sleep do to you?

But, it doesn't have to be this way. You may need to weather the storm for a period of time, but by steadily developing the right habits, you can reboot your recovery and rediscover your best health.

Why Am I Always Sick in Mid Life?

Parents with young children at home are often sick. This is not breaking news. And while it's true that kids in nursery or daycare and schools are exposed to more pathogens (and thus you are as well), it's not the primary reason you're always getting sick.

In order to get sick, two things must happen; you must be exposed to a virus *and* you must be immune-compromised. While you may not have much control over the former, you certainly do over the latter. It starts with sleep. The importance of sleep for maintaining a robust immune system was first highlighted by a study comparing how much sleep you get nightly with your risk of infection. Researchers divided the groups into varying sleep times – more than 7 hours, 6–7 hours, and less than 6 hours per night – to see who got sick the most. How did lack of sleep impact infection? The group getting between 6–7 hours a night were three times more likely to get sick (compared to those with at least 7 hours nightly), while the group getting less than 6 hours' sleep were at a 4.5-fold increased risk of infection.[8]

Don't Reach for the Coffee Immediately

After all those restless nights, the first thing you probably reach for is your morning cup of coffee, right? Well, caffeine after a poor night's sleep might not be the best idea.

In 2020, a study in the *British Journal of Nutrition* by the Centre for Nutrition, Exercise and Metabolism in the UK, examined how a morning coffee impacts markers of metabolic health after a night of broken sleep. By itself, a night of bad sleep does little to impact your metabolism adversely. But, when you rely on caffeine too heavily the following morning, it can really throw your blood sugar levels out of whack.

Study participants who drank a strong black coffee before breakfast exhibited a 50 per cent greater blood glucose response to breakfast.[9] That is a massive spike. But, there is an easy fix. If you eat breakfast first, then have your coffee, you offset these effects. (Breathe a sigh of relief!)

Can You 'Bank' Sleep?

If you know you're about to go through an intense period of lack of sleep, is it possible to offset the adverse effects on mental and physical performance by 'banking' more sleep in the days leading up to it? Researchers extended the sleep of 12 adults over a six-day period before one night of total sleep deprivation. Mental and physical performance measures were assessed before and after the sleepless night. What did they uncover? Adding an extra 2 hours' sleep per night, over the six days, significantly improved time to exhaustion in the exercise test (reducing how difficult the task felt to participants) and positively impacted mental performance as well.[10] The study authors also noted that banking sleep could be highly beneficial for individuals with a high workload and young children. Can't find an extra 2 hours to nudge forward your bedtime? You're not alone. But, even 30–60 minutes can have highly beneficial effects.

While 'banking' sleep can be helpful at specific times, most people still need more sleep *all* the time. Dr Norah Simpson, PhD, from Stanford University School of Medicine says that repeatedly trying to offset lack of sleep during the week by catching up on your sleep over the weekend is not a recipe for long-term success. She advises focusing on your sleep on a night-to-night basis, rather than running really lean during the week and hoping to catch up on weekends, because of the myriad negative effects on mental health and performance, such as diminished attention, learning, ability to problem-solve and mood.[11] There is also a genetic component to how sleep deprivation impacts you. Your vulnerability to sleep loss appears to be an inherent trait, so if you really struggle on short sleep, it may be difficult to offset by merely banking sleep and you'll need to be consistent with your efforts to commit to better nightly sleep.[12]

The Sleep and Immunity Connection: How to Prevent and Recover from Cold and Flu

Sleep and immunity are intertwined and being short of sleep in mid life puts you at an increased risk of infection, cold and flu. These supplements can act as preventative strategies to reduce the duration and severity of such illnesses.

Vitamin D

Incredibly, approximately 5 per cent of your entire human genome is impacted by vitamin D. If your vitamin D levels are low, you're at greater risk of colds and flu.[13] Moreover, the lower your

Nap If You Need To

If you can't increase your total nightly sleep time, due to work or family commitments, aim to increase your *weekly* total sleep by adding short naps.

Naps are best done in 30- or 90-minute 'sleep opportunities', meaning you set the alarm on your phone for this amount of time. Next, place a mask over your eyes, put on some relaxing music or white noise, and lie down. For short power naps, you may not fall asleep and that's okay. But these short rest periods are still highly beneficial to the sleep-deprived, mid-life brain, increasing alpha brainwave activity to support better cognition.

For longer naps, you will fall asleep, so be sure to wake up no later than 4pm. Ideally, naps should be taken between 1–4pm and the earlier you rise in the morning, the earlier your nap time should be in that time frame. Adding to your weekly sleep total via naps is a great way to augment recovery.

vitamin D status, the worse your symptoms are likely to be and the more days you're likely to struggle with symptoms. But, the good news is that higher levels of vitamin D in winter and spring are associated with reduced frequency of infections.[14] Aim to supplement with 2,000–4,000 IU vitamin D during the winter months to maintain levels above 90nmol/L (36ng/mL), and if immunity is a high concern, aim to keep levels above 120nmol/L (48ng/mL).

Step 3 - Upgrade Your Sleep

Sleep science and education have come a long way in the last decade. Recovery expert Dr Shona Halson, PhD, at the Australian Institute for Sport, is quick to point out that it's the application of sleep science we really need to focus on now.

Where most people fall short is setting up a sleep routine. You must create the environment and behaviours to help you unwind at the end of the day (without half a bottle of red wine!), so you can maximize your ability to recharge for the next day.

Commit to a Sleep Routine

Humans are creatures of habit. If you use your phone as an alarm clock, you'll likely scroll your Twitter or Instagram feed before bed. Bad idea. The typical mid-life adult aged 35–44 checks their phone about 35 times per day or approximately every 12 minutes. When this becomes a pattern before bedtime, it's a big problem for sleep and recovery. One hour before bed, turn off all social media and power down your laptop to give your (overly taxed) nervous system the chance to unwind. The key action to start this process is putting your phone away. Put. Your. Phone. Away. Go 'old school' and get yourself an alarm clock because taking your phone, or tablet, into the bedroom at night sets the wrong pattern for deep, restful sleep.

Sleep scientists have also recently discovered that your body naturally dials down inflammation while you sleep (during dark hours), but if you're exposed to constant light from devices or staying up too late, it leads to a greater output of pro-inflammatory markers.[15]

Once the shackles of technology are removed, you may notice a wave of anxiety, but don't worry, it will pass. What can you do to decompress? Read for pleasure, watch something relaxing on TV (not your tablet), do some light stretching, go for a walk, meditate, take a hot bath or shower, plan out your next day with a pen and notebook, talk to your partner. Your brain and body need time to shift from fifth gear back down to first. Remember, the missing link to recovery is *actually* commiting to it; aim for five nights of good sleep per week. (Go to DrBubbs.com /PEAK40 to download your Sleep Routine blueprint.)

Sleep Total and Timing

If you're not achieving at least 7 hours, increase your sleep total by half an hour (every week) until you get to the minimum. From there, continue to nudge up another 30 minutes to 7.5–8 hours' per night, up to a maximum of 8–9 hours.

Anchoring your wake time – when you get up – is the key to getting your sleep back on point. If you struggle with sleep and get up at varying hours every day, start to lock in a consistent time instead.

Limit Sleep Saboteurs

Caffeine is a potent sleep saboteur. Too much caffeine in the afternoon or, worse, the evening, can delay sleep onset and reduce your total sleep time and quality. Aim to keep your caffeine consumption to before noon or 1pm. (If you use a pre-workout formula, be sure to check if it contains caffeine.)

Alcohol is another major sleep saboteur. Alcohol is a nervine, meaning it relaxes your nervous system. That's why you may feel that 'aah' moment when you take the first sip of that glass of wine after a long day or putting the kids to bed, but scientists have identified alcohol as one of the most powerful suppressors of REM sleep, the crucial recovery time when your brain is synthesizing and consolidating new information. When you drink alcohol too late in the evening, your liver begins to metabolize the ingested alcohol and increases your core body temperature as a result. This is a problem for quality sleep because your body temperature is supposed to drop at night to support deep and restful sleep. The increase in body temperature ultimately impairs your sleep architecture and quality of rest. Alcohol also taxes your nervous system, which if you've ever used a sleep-monitoring device, you'll see as your heart rate increasing by 10–20 beats per minute after having a glass or two of wine before bed. How much alcohol *can* you consume? If you're looking to improve health or lose weight, your goal should be to eliminate alcohol at least four nights per week. What about the other three nights? One to two glasses are fine (ok, ok ... one of those nights you can have three!).

Sleep apnea (when breathing is interrupted during sleep) also hinders quality sleep and weight gain is the primary culprit. Research shows that the larger a person's BMI or neck circumference, the higher their risk of sleep apnea.[16] If you're an endurance enthusiast, you may suffer from restless legs syndrome, another medical condition that can impair sleep.[17]

Supplemental Sleep Support

Sometimes in mid life, the brain and body need a little nudge in the right direction to support a deeper sleep. Melatonin helps to regulate the timing of your sleep, signalling to your brain that it's time to begin the recovery process. If you're a 'night owl', who naturally prefers to go to bed later but can't due to work and life demands, melatonin may be particularly helpful. The medical term for this is delayed sleep-wake phase disorder (DSWPD) and is defined as a circadian rhythm disorder in which your sleep schedule is shifted later into the night. Research shows low doses of melatonin taken before the desired bedtime can help people with DSWPD adjust their sleep cycle forward.[18]

What about if you're simply looking to improve your sleep? The American Academy of Sleep

Medicine (AASM) says there isn't sufficient scientific evidence to support the use of melatonin in reducing insomnia. However, some sleep experts point to evidence that melatonin can help people who struggle to fall asleep.[19] In my experience, a low dose of 0.5–1.5mg of melatonin per night for a month can be a nice way to test-drive whether it improves your sleep and recovery (melatonin sprays or time-release capsules seem to work best).

Vitamin C

Vitamin C is a potent, water-soluble antioxidant and it plays a key role in immune function. It's found in high concentration in white blood cells, but when you get sick, levels fall dramatically. If you start to feel rundown, research shows a daily dose of 200mg of vitamin C can help protect you against the common cold.[20] If you're exercising intensely, recent trials in recreational athletes and the military found 1,000mg per day of vitamin C reduced the incidence of common colds by as much as 52 per cent.[21] Already sick? No problem. Supplementing with vitamin C during illness helps to improve immune function by mitigating against excessive tissue damage. Try ramping up your vitamin C intake to 3,000–6,000mg on the first day of infection.[22]

Probiotics

Your gut and immune system are intricately linked, with over 70 per cent of your immune system located in your gut. Does that translate to a potential therapeutic role for probiotics on immunity? A recent systematic review of 20 placebo-controlled studies found probiotic supplementation was able to reduce the number of sick days and shorten the length of illness.[23] Another major review found that probiotics reduced cold and flu by 47 per cent and cut short the average duration of illness by 2 days.[24] Aim for multi-strain formulas that contain 10^{10} live bacteria per capsule of *Lactobacillus* or *Bifidobacterium* strains.

Zinc Lozenges

Zinc lozenges are a quick, convenient and evidence-based solution for reducing the duration of common colds when taken within 24 hours of symptoms starting.[25] Zinc lozenges also help to target the nasal epithelium to reduce inflammation. Aim for 75mg of zinc acetate or zinc gluconate lozenges divided throughout the day.

———

In 2010, while preparing for the upcoming London Olympic Games, Radcliffe noted she was very fortunate that her young daughter had slept through the night from a very young age, allowing her to get the rest she needed to train and recover. It was even more important for her in mid life, when most marathon runners had retired, to maximize every possible marginal gain. In 2011, three years after her last win at a major marathon and after the birth of her second child, Radcliffe finished third at the Berlin Marathon, qualifying for the London 2012 Olympic Games at the age of 37, an incredible accomplishment in mid life.

CHAPTER 11

Recovery Strategies

'Pain is a more terrible lord of mankind than even death itself.'
— **ALBERT SCHWEITZER**, medical missionary
and Nobel Peace Prize winner

The day after competing in the final round of the US Open in 2010, Phil Mickelson woke up in crippling pain. He couldn't move; he couldn't even get out of bed. Mickelson is one of the greatest golfers in today's game, winner of five major championships and future Hall of Famer. But that morning, all Mickelson worried about was being able to move again, pain free. A visit to his doctor, and then a specialist rheumatologist, led to a diagnosis of psoriatic arthritis. Psoriatic arthritis is an autoimmune condition, where the body's immune system begins attacking itself (in Mickelson's case specifically the joints), like 'friendly fire' from your body's own immune system army. Medication dramatically improved Mickelson's condition but, years later, he still wasn't all the way back to his dominant form and hadn't won another major. By Mickelson's admission, his poor diet, lack of exercise and weight gain were all worsening his condition.

Autoimmune conditions like psoriatic arthritis have strong links to your digestive system, where over 70 per cent of your immune system is located. Mickelson's poor food choices led to weight gain, which is known to dramatically shift the balance of bacteria in the gut, exaggerating the inflammatory process and scrambling the immune system response. The medication helped to reduce Mickelson's chronic inflammation, but it didn't resolve all the pain. It couldn't offset Mickelson's poor diet and lack of fitness. Two years after his diagnosis, Mickelson decided it was time to focus on his diet and exercise regime.

Rebuild and Recover

Do you grunt or groan when getting out of bed in the morning? Does it take you a while to shake off the stiffness and achiness? Do constant pain, discomfort and inflammation derail your day before it even gets started? Chronic pain impacts your movement, your work and even your mood. When you're in pain, all you can think about is your pain.

Managing Chronic Pain

In the last chapter, you learned that if you lack sleep, you're more likely to struggle with pain and injury (not to mention weight gain). Improving blood glucose control, losing weight and rebuilding your fitness are key fundamentals to reducing the inflammatory noise in your body leading to pain.[1] Once you have tackled those three elements, you can begin to explore the more marginal gains at the top of the recovery pyramid – recovery strategies to reduce pain and discomfort in the short-term and set yourself up for pain-free living in the long run.

The Arctic Advantage:
Ice Baths and Cold Plunges

Hydrotherapy, the application of hot or cold water, has been prescribed as a treatment for chronic conditions and improving vitality since the time of Ancient Greece (and likely earlier in the East). The godfather of modern medicine, Hippocrates, routinely used cold-water treatments for chronic conditions.[2] In Roman times, bathing was centred around the practice of relaxing in a series of heated rooms before finishing off with a cold plunge at the end.[3] Throughout our evolution, humans have been exposed to very cold (or very hot) temperatures. Today's climate-controlled world is nice (and comfortable) but the lack of exposure to the natural elements – hardwired into our DNA through millions of years of evolution – may be making us more fragile and less resilient.

Jumping into cold water has a profound impact on your physiology, both physically and mentally. So much so, it appears it may even boost mood and improve your resilience to stress in other areas of your life. Professor Mike Tipton, an environmental physiologist at the University of Portsmouth in the UK, has found in his research that there are two distinct mechanisms at play when you're exposed to low temperatures.[4] The first is the initial shock of plunging into very cold waters: your heart rate immediately ramps up, your respiratory rate quickens and you can feel the adrenaline pumping in your body. Your brain gets a surge of endorphins, you can get an emotional lift and your cortisol stress hormones ramp up, reducing the sensation of pain. You are experiencing a very primal 'fight or flight' response.

The second is how your body adapts in the longer term after repeated exposures to cold-water plunges, and Tipton and his team have noted that the more exposures you get, the lesser the 'fight or flight' response appears to be. The spike in heart rate and respiration rates seen in study participants fell by as much as 50 per cent after six exposures.[5] Interestingly, this adaptive response may provide a crossover benefit in your ability to cope with other stressors in your life.

Cross-Over Benefits

Ice baths and cold tubs have been used in sport for decades, yet the study of ice baths (referred to as cold-water immersion or CWI in the research) has only recently exploded over the past half-decade. Scientists are still trying to uncover how (and why) it may support recovery. Cold-water immersion has a big impact on your nervous system, but not the expected one. The initial blast to your nervous system leads to a reduction in nerve conduction velocity and inhibits pain receptor sensitivity, thereby producing an anesthetic effect and reducing your sensation of pain.[6] This is good news for chronic pain sufferers. The potential threat of freezing cold water lights up your brain, down-regulating pain sensation and other areas of discomfort. The reduction in pain you experience in cold water, combined with your ability to move your limbs (without inducing pain), dials down long-standing pain pathways in the brain, a little bit like rebooting your computer.[7]

Cold Tubs: Reducing Muscle Soreness

To recover effectively from exercise, your muscles, ligaments and tissues need nutrients. Nutrients are delivered around the body via blood flow, a key reason why light exercise is used as a recovery strategy in elite and professional sports after intense training days or games. But it's not just light exercise that improves blood flow, you can also achieve it passively, by sitting in very cold (or very hot) water.

Ice baths have been shown to reduce muscle soreness and markers of muscle damage in athletes after sprints on a bike or in a simulated team sport game for up to 96 hours (4 days).[8] The major advantage from cold-water immersion appears to be a quicker recovery of your faster-twitch muscle fibres (the more explosive ones needed for sprinting and jumping). This is a great strategy when you're trying to optimize recovery, like during a competition or the gruelling competitive season for an athlete.

When you think of cold-water recovery, you often think of American football or rugby players seated in giant tubs of ice after an intense training session. But, what about after your typical training session? Do ice baths help you to recover more efficiently? Not exactly. Ice baths after training can actually blunt some of the benefits of your training session. A randomized study of an eight-week training block compared the effects of cold-water immersion versus passive rest (the control). Researchers investigated how the cold-water immersions would impact performance on a 1-repetition maximum leg press (i.e. the maximum amount of weight you could lift) and jump performance. What did they find? When comparing pre- versus post-study performance, the cold-water immersion group experienced a moderate negative effect on both exercises, as well as a larger negative impact on muscle thickness.[9] While ice baths have been staples in athletic training for decades, new science is continuing to uncover that it's not beneficial directly after a training session. If you're an exercise enthusiast training for a marathon, triathlon, cycling event, Crossfit or the like, this simply means you should not have your cold bath or plunge directly after training, but later in the day (or first thing in the morning – that will definitely get you going!).

Cold Plunge to Ramp Up Resilience

How does a cold plunge or ice bath possibly increase your resilience to other stressors? (An important question in mid life, when stressors are abundant and intense!) Scientists call it cross adaptation; the better you adapt to one stressor, the more likely you are to get a crossover benefit to other stressors. For example, research on individuals adapted to cold plunges shows they acclimatize more quickly to simulated high altitude (low oxygen) settings when compared to those who are not.[10] The biggest win in mid life may be how physical stress adaptations may transfer over to mental stress adaptations. How? Your nervous system is

Are You Ready for the Plunge?

Do you have a river, lake, ocean or sea nearby? Ground-breaking research shows there is even more benefit to a cold plunge when it takes place in nature, which is caused by the psychological effects of just being outdoors.[11]

SAFETY NOTE: If you are doing a cold plunge in nature or a pool, always go with a buddy (never on your own). Consult your doctor first if you have a medical condition or are in poor health.

under a heavy load due to the constant crying of a baby, lack of sleep, demanding boss, and the like. It is constantly stuck in the 'on' state. The exposure to a massive stress response, like a cold plunge, hits the 'off' button. It provides such an overwhelming signal to the brain that it helps to dampen your stress response to life's (non-life-threatening) hurdles. All of a sudden, your brain perceives life's many little stresses as just that. Note, though, that a cold shower doesn't have the same effect as sitting submerged in cold water.

Cold plunges may even be able to improve your mental health as well. Low mood and depression have been tightly linked to chronically high levels of inflammation. Persistently elevated blood sugar levels and weight gain are principal drivers of inflammation, along with lack of sleep. When you're sleep-deprived, you tend to reach for more processed food, continuing to exacerbate the inflammatory loop. Exercise is a

Cryotherapy for Recovery: Is It Worth the Expense?

Cryotherapy is the latest buzzword in recovery. Whole body cryotherapy (WBC) is like something out of *Star Trek*: you stand in a tank up to your neck and freezing cold temperatures (−80 to −190°C/−112 to −310°F) are blasted over your body for 2–4 minutes. Cryotherapy is said to be beneficial for reducing inflammation, muscle damage and muscle soreness after exercise. What does the research say? The best results from cryotherapy are seen when it's used repeatedly over multiple days; studies showing three and five sessions of cryotherapy encouraged faster recovery in muscle function and reduced pain perceptions.[12] But, there are some significant limitations. A major selling point is the incredibly cold temperatures the body is exposed to, which make it seem better than an ice bath. Yet, when you compare a cold bath at 8°C (46°F) versus a cryotherapy session at −110°C (−166°F), both elicit the same effect on core body temperature. How is this possible? Air has poor thermal conductivity compared to water and thus prevents significant cooling of subcutaneous and core tissues. In short, cryotherapy definitely makes your skin a lot colder, but this effect dissipates after 1 hour; a faster return to baseline than cold-water baths.[13] Also, when compared head-to-head as a recovery tool, cold-water immersions are superior to cryotherapy.[14] To sum up, cold tubs are a better (and much cheaper) bet.

powerful anti-inflammatory stimulus, but, of course, in mid life it's harder to carve out time for it. How do cold plunges fit into this mix? A cold plunge provides an instant spark to help cool the pro-inflammatory process. You also get an endorphin rush; you feel better, you sleep better and, thus, you make better food choices. One small change, like taking a cold plunge, can make other habits more enticing (and easier) to adhere to, ultimately impacting many areas of your life positively.

How Long to Cold Plunge?

Ready to test-drive a cold plunge? You're probably wondering how long you need to endure the arctic temperatures? Studies have seen benefits with as little as 3 minutes to as long as 20 minutes in waist- to shoulder-height water. Recovery expert Dr Shona Halson, PhD, highlights that, based on the research, the 'sweet spot' appears to be approximately 11–15 minutes at 11–15°C (51.8–59°F).[15]

Bring on the Heat: Hot Tubs and Saunas

Of course, the challenge with cold plunges and ice baths is actually getting people to do it. For some, cold plunges might be too wide a gap to navigate. Interestingly, there is a more comfortable option. Both cold- and hot-water immersions are effective at reducing symptoms of joint pain, arthritis or fibromyalgia, as well as aiding the recovery post-traumatic injury.[16] Perhaps for some people, a better place to start might be a hot bath (keeping, if you can, the temperature at 38–40°C/100–104°F for 11–15 minutes).

Research shows hot-water immersion (HWI) can reduce markers of inflammation and protect you against cardiovascular disease.[17] For example, hot-water immersions have been found to be effective for improving blood flow and cardiovascular function in patients with congestive heart failure. It does so via the effect of dilating blood vessels, which subsequently leads to an increase in cardiac output, where your body must respond and adapt to maintain blood flow through the dilated vessels.[18] In short, in hot water your body needs to pump more blood to maintain the same pressure.

Heat for Glucose Control

Hot baths are also a powerful (and enjoyable) tool for improving your glucose control, lowering fasting glucose, insulin and HbA1c levels in as little as 2–3 weeks.[19] Hot-water immersion is such a potent therapy, it's been suggested as an alternative to exercise to improve metabolic health in people who are unable to exercise. How does a hot tub work for glucose control? When you submerge yourself into a steaming hot bath, the increase in body temperature increases the glucose uptake into your muscles, a big win for blood sugar control.[20] From a recovery standpoint, studies show hot baths increase blood flow 3- to 4-fold to the lower body, which is crucial for recovery.[21] Hot baths, or contrasting hot with cold, are used extensively in elite and pro sports to support athlete recovery.[22]

Hot-water immersion can also benefit fatigue and depression. Regular hot tubs or hot sauna use have been shown to elicit key physiological responses that improve symptoms of low energy and low mood.[23]

How Long to Hot Tub?

The time commitment is similar to cold plunges: aim for 11–15 minutes at temperatures between 38–40°C (100–104°F).[24] This is most easily achieved in a hot tub, but can be achieved at home in your bath (you'll just need to continuously top up with hot water to keep the temperature elevated throughout the prescribed time).

Always ensure you're well-hydrated first (a simple urine dip-stick test is cheap to purchase online) and remember to take your time getting out (so as not to feel light-headed), and if you feel it's too hot or you don't feel right, get out.

Nutrition Strategies to Reduce Pain and Muscle Damage

Why in mid life does it feel as if, even after an easy workout, you struggle with more pain and discomfort? The scientific term is exercise-induced muscle damage (EIMD) and it's characterized by symptoms that come on directly after training and can persist for 1–5 days afterwards. What happens if muscle damage is too exaggerated after a workout? It impacts on how well you move, how sore you are, your range of motion and muscle capacity to produce force.[25] You need to be patient and build slowly. If you haven't had the time to train or if you exercise only sporadically, you can't dive right into the deep end all at once.

Protein

As we've seen, protein is crucial to muscular repair, recovery and rebuilding after resistance and endurance exercise. It also plays a key role in reducing important markers of muscle damage so you can exercise daily without feeling too stiff or too sore.[26] It's a major reason why *Set Your Protein* is a fundamental pillar for success. It sets you up to exercise and recover effectively, as well as providing the building blocks to keep your joints healthy and strong. The addition of 'portable nutrition' to your diet, in the form of a protein shake, can help to reduce muscle damage post-exercise. Aim for 20–40g whey isolate or plant-based protein after exercise, or as your mid-afternoon snack.

Vitamin D

Vitamin D has a potent impact on exercise recovery via its effect on satellite cell activity. Satellite cells are activated after exercise and sustained activation provides your muscles with an enhanced capacity to adapt more effectively from training.[27] Vitamin D supports satellite cell activation and thus plays a key role in mitigating exercise-induced muscle damage. For example, runners with low vitamin D exhibited increased inflammatory responses post-exercise, compared to runners with higher vitamin D, who experienced an anti-inflammatory response.[28]

A sedentary lifestyle, or working primarily indoors, can lead to a lack of sufficient sun exposure and subsequent vitamin D deficiency (less than 12mg/dL or 30nmol/L). But it's not just lack of sun that sabotages vitamin D status. If you're struggling with weight gain, high sugar levels, high blood pressure or a chronic health condition, your levels are probably insufficient or deficient. Aim to supplement with 2,000 IU per day to ensure you keep blood levels of vitamin D above 30mg/dL (75nmol/L).

Creatine

Creatine plays a key role in recovery as it has specific beneficial effects on satellite cell numbers and muscle function post-training.[29] Creatine is an especially potent recovery supplement because creatine-rich foods, like herring, beef and other animal proteins, cannot augment creatine stores to the same degree as supplementation. Aim for 3g and 5g daily for women and men, respectively.

Omega-3

Omega-3 polyunsaturated fats, specifically eicosapentaenoic acid (EPA) and docosahexaenoic acid (DHA), are also important nutrients that exert powerful anti-inflammatory effects. Numerous

Table 11.1. Supplements for Recovery from Exercise

Supplement	Dose
Protein	20–40g
Vitamin D	2,000 IU/day
Creatine	3g for women 5g for men
Omega-3 (combined EPA/DHA)	1,100–1,500mg

studies have shown beneficial effects of omega-3 supplementation on inflammation, oxidative stress and muscle function after intense exercise.[30] Aim for a dose of 1,100–1,500mg (combined EPA/DHA) in the hours after exercise (or at dinner time) to support recovery.

———

When Phil Mickelson was diagnosed with psoriatic arthritis in 2010 at the age of 40, his game had derailed. He had previously won four major championships but was desperately seeking to add the British and US Opens to his résumé. Phil's desire to sustain peak performance in mid life ignited his motivation to change his diet and exercise regime to support better recovery and therefore performance. How did it work out for him? Three years later, after making significant changes to his diet, Mickelson accomplished a lifelong goal of winning the British Open at the historic Muirfield golf club in Scotland. Mickelson said of his performance, 'I played arguably the best round of my career, and shot the round of my life.'[31] Fast forward to today and Mickelson has been quoted as saying, 'I ended up eating poorly, I ended up drinking soda, I ended up eating sugar – I just didn't eat the way

I should have and I think it led to me getting psoriatic arthritis, and I think it led to me not being overall healthy.'[32]

Mickelson has shown that PEAK40 performance is indeed possible! In what area of your health and performance would you like to see a personal best? Apply the principles. Stay consistent. And with the right mindset, you can achieve it.

Unlock Your Potential

CHAPTER 12

Traits, Values and Skills

'Knowing others is wisdom;
Knowing yourself is enlightenment.'

— LAO TZU, Chinese philosopher and writer

E rling Kagge is an explorer. He is the first person in history to reach the 'three poles' – North Pole, South Pole and the summit of Mount Everest. During these long and arduous treks, Kagge experienced extreme periods of silence; the longest of which was 50 days. During these extended periods, he realized, as he so eloquently describes in his appropriately named bestselling book *Silence: In the Age of Noise*, that he had a primal need for silence.

Today, it is increasingly difficult to find space and moments of silence; to just be. In order to achieve your goals, you need to change some of your behaviours, and while this may seem like an analytical problem (i.e. understanding logically what needs to be done), it's actually a far deeper and more emotional experience. To successfully change behaviours, you need to understand yourself. But, if you're too busy or distracted in today's attention economy (where attention has been commodified by social media) to reflect on yourself and your values, and how your actions align with those values, you'll likely be frustrated with the results.

A common theme when clients struggle to achieve goals is to look outwards – a new diet regime, a new exercise plan, a new coach, and the like. More often than not, the real answers are found within. When asked how he was able to complete the arduous 50-day trek across the South Pole in temperatures as low as −50°C/−58°F, Kagge replied matter-of-factly, 'You put one foot in front of the other ... and do it enough times.' It's beautifully simple, yet ruthlessly effective.

Solving complex problems like a chronic health condition, weight gain or low mood requires a similar mindset. Success is best measured in elite sport or in behaviour change by trying simply to 'win the day'. Not yesterday, not tomorrow, but the day that's right in front of you. You must block out the external noise of social media, advice from friends, and the like, and keep yourself grounded in the present. Finding a moment's silence to look within, to reflect, to observe, is a key part of the process. Nature provides an escape from the noise; an endless expanse of snow, a vast ocean or an imposing forest. In that silence, there is an opportunity to explore; to know yourself better. To develop the mindset skills to overcome the hurdles and challenges of mid life and beyond.

Understanding Yourself

Do you know yourself? I mean, do you *really* know yourself? Not just the obvious personality traits you like (or dislike), but the more subtle factors operating under the surface. Understanding your personality is important not only for the relationships in your life, your work or your performance goals, but also for overcoming challenges that present themselves in these domains. Are certain personality traits part of the roadblock? Personality traits are like the hardware on your computer, deeply embedded and built-in. It takes a very long time (if ever) to change personality traits. In this context, that shouldn't be your goal. The objective here is to understand your personality so you can identify possible blind spots, which may be contributing to behaviours that are holding you back (without you even realizing it).

You're probably familiar with the Big 5 Personality Traits: openness, conscientiousness, extraversion, agreeableness and neuroticism (the acronym is ocean). Openness to experience includes aspects like intellectual curiosity and creativity. Conscientiousness refers to how well you're organized, responsible and productive. Extraversion is just as it sounds – are you sociable and assertive, or more reserved and passive. Agreeableness encompasses aspects like compassion, respectfulness and trust in others, while neuroticism describes one's tendency towards anxiety and depression.

For example, the more competitive you are, the more likely you are to be disagreeable (to some degree). Individuals with competitive/disagreeable character traits tend to be tough, straightforward and aggressive. When performance is going well, your competitive edge pushes you to new heights. But when you're stuck (and you're probably not used to being stuck), the disagreeable factor sabotages your success because you struggle to heed the advice of coaches or take solace in the comfort of friends or family. People who score higher in neuroticism are much more likely to experience anxiety and emotional pain. This can lead to strong emotional responses when goals aren't being met and the focus is too far into the future, which makes the objective seem as realistic as climbing Mount Everest. If you have the self-awareness to appreciate this is a tendency for you, an ability to let these emotions pass before making any key decisions is very helpful for long-term success.

Working with Your Personality

Where do you fit on the continuums? Each of the personality traits reflects patterns in how you think and feel (and therefore behave). Understanding yourself is a crucial piece of the puzzle. You're not going to change your personality (or somebody else's, for that matter), but the process of understanding your

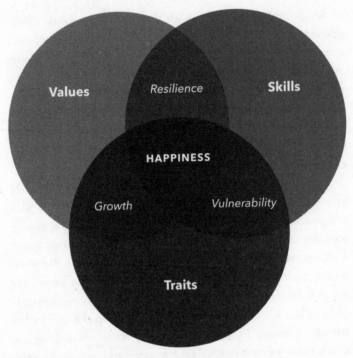

Figure 12.1. Traits, values and skills.

personality provides you with perspective and can help illuminate the right path to success. (Interested to understand your personality? You can find a Big 5 questionnaire online.)

To help understand how personality traits fit into the paradigm of your values and mindset skills, see Figure 12.1. The intersection of these domains is where growth, resilience, vulnerability and, ultimately, happiness occur. Let's now explore your values.

What Really Motivates You?

Your values are the fundamental beliefs that guide and motivate you and your actions. They're the things you believe to be important about how you live and how you work. Your values are the motivation behind *purposeful* action. They orient you towards your ultimate goals. Have you ever taken the time, really taken the time, to reflect on your core values?

Why are values important for supporting behaviour change? Have you ever tried to 'tell yourself' what to do? You say, 'I'm going to stop snacking at night', and after two days you're back to your old ways. You tell yourself, 'I'm going to exercise every morning,' and after a week you're back to hitting snooze.

It's difficult to 'tell yourself' to do things. You start out on your new plan riding the wave of inspiration in the first week, achieving your targets and feeling fulfilled, but as the tide moves out and the wave of inspiration subsides, you struggle to maintain the same gusto. The hard truth is that most of us have little control over our attentional focus; it's a skill we must develop. Behaviour change takes time.

You Are Led by Your Values

If you aren't aware of your values, it's much more difficult to develop a new habit. Bryce Tully, MSc, Mental Performance Coach of the Canadian Women's National Basketball Team, puts this into perspective stating, 'Everything is a rule until people know why.'[1] That diet you're following has rules. The exercise plan, more rules. It's okay to follow rules (especially in the short-term), but they are just rules. Until you can connect how each rule aligns with your values, you struggle to achieve long-term compliance (from yourself or from a client). For example, Tully recently shared a story about a competition that the women's national team took part in a few years ago. The coaches wanted all the players to wear their national team tracksuits on the bus, on the way to the venue. While it's normal for all the players to come out on to the court in their team gear, wearing it on the bus up to that point had been optional. Many players preferred to wear more comfortable clothing en route to the game. However, one particular coach was adamant they should be worn on the bus and was frustrated at the lack of pride the team was showing. On the other hand, the players were also annoyed; they wondered why they couldn't just wear the items they preferred and were used to. At Tully's suggestion, the coach decided to address the team and share his story of making the national team and wearing the jersey himself, and how they would've had to tear it away from him, he was so proud to be wearing it. Once the players understood why it mattered, the behaviour change was straightforward. Their values aligned with his – they were proud to be representing their country. When values align, great things can happen.

What Are Your Core Values?

Try this exercise. From the list of Top 99 Values (see Table 12.1), narrow it down to your top 10. Next, review your top 10 and taper it down to three. Lastly, write out a few sentences or a paragraph about why these values matter to you (and include the words you selected). The exercise is an enlightening one and will highlight the direction you should be orienting your life. Of course, not all your actions will be in alignment with your values. You will have blind spots; behaviours you don't realize are in opposition and that are incongruent with your values.

Why does this matter? If you want to resolve complex problems, like weight gain, a chronic health condition and low mood, you'll need to successfully change current behaviours. You dramatically increase your odds of success if you can attach the new behaviour to your values. For example, if family time is an important value for you, yet weight gain leads to low energy levels and low mood, it will adversely impact your ability to spend quality time with your family, leaving you frustrated that

Table 12.1. Top 99 Values

Accountability	Fitness	Preparedness
Achievement	Focus	Professionalism
Adventurousness	Freedom	Prudence
Ambition	Fun	Reliability
Assertiveness	Generosity	Resourcefulness
Balance	Goodness	Restraint
Belonging	Grace	Rigor
Boldness	Growth	Security
Calmness	Happiness	Self-actualization
Commitment	Hard work	Self-control
Compassion	Health	Selflessness
Competitiveness	Honesty	Sensitivity
Consistency	Honour	Spontaneity
Contentment	Humility	Stability
Control	Independence	Strength
Cooperation	Inquisitiveness	Structure
Creativity	Insightfulness	Success
Curiosity	Intelligence	Support
Dependability	Intuition	Talent
Determination	Joy	Teamwork
Discipline	Justice	Thankfulness
Dynamism	Leadership	Thoroughness
Efficiency	Legacy	Thoughtfulness
Empathy	Love	Tolerance
Enthusiasm	Loyalty	Traditionalism
Equality	Making a difference	Trustworthiness
Excellence	Mastery	Truth-seeking
Excitement	Merit	Understanding
Exploration	Openness	Uniqueness
Expressiveness	Order	Unity
Fairness	Originality	Usefulness
Faith	Perfection	Vision
Family-oriented	Positivity	Vitality

you can't achieve your goal. Once you shine a light and become aware of your values, you realize that changing your nutrition behaviour – for example, not snacking late at night – is not really about weight loss, but rather about improving the experience you have when spending time with your family. Having clear values fans the flames of behaviour change towards the intended target.

Mindset – Build 'Trainable' Skills

If your personality traits are the hardware on your computer and values are the coding, your mindset skills are the software that holds your values in place. Mindset skills, for example mindfulness (the ability to maintain attention), self-talk and optimism, are trainable, unlike personality traits. When you upgrade your mental performance skillset, it allows you to direct your actions and behaviours more effectively towards your values and, ultimately, your goals. You don't have to listen to your inner monologue berating you for not waking up early to run, snacking too frequently, or generally not living up to your expectations; you have the power to code new, positive thought patterns. Developing mindset skills orients you towards your values, empowering you to navigate challenging situations (where coming up against roadblocks is inevitable). Invest the time in developing them, to rewrite your mindset software, and you'll amplify your odds of success. Building these skills are a good starting point:

- Self-talk (confidence)
- Mindfulness (ability to maintain attention)
- Optimism (positivity)

Self-Talk

Why do you remember the bad things that happen in your day more clearly than the good? Why do you remember the negative comment from a friend or colleague weeks, months, even years later, but the positive ones seem to slip past? Because you're human. In evolutionary terms, we're hard-wired to default to negative, cautious or fearful thoughts, in order to survive. Hundreds of thousands of years ago, if you heard a snarl in the night, it was far more advantageous to err on the side of caution, than it was to put yourself in harm's way. If you got it wrong, you were dead. Today, this evolutionary hangover is still within us.

Self-talk reverberates deep in your subconscious and negative self-talk is like a heavy backpack weighing you down, quickly sabotaging your mood, confidence and likelihood of success, and preventing you from moving forwards at speed. When you add to the mix the effect that lack of sleep and chronic stress have on triggering overly emotional responses and preventing you from thinking 'big picture', it's easy to see how self-talk can quickly turn south (and your confidence along with it).

Building Confidence

Where does confidence come from? It comes from preparation, hard work and past successes. If you enter a new domain or haven't succeeded in a current one for some time, how do you cultivate the confidence to enter the arena, to be willing to put yourself out there and try? You need to rewire your internal monologue.

The godfather of modern psychology, Albert Ellis, uncovered that how you talk to yourself, and think to yourself, about your experiences has a major influence on how you perceive them.[2] Thoughts like 'This is too hard, I can't do it' or 'I'll never be good enough' or 'This won't work for me', leave you in an anxious or worried state. Your thoughts are tightly linked to your emotions, making negative self-talk a major PEAK40 health and performance roadblock. This is even more true in domains where you've struggled in the past.

The language you use to describe your situation, in life, at work, or in performance goals, determines how you actually see it, experience it and participate in it. These were the findings of renowned professor Will Hart, PhD, from the University of Alabama, who proved positive self-talk to be an effective strategy for boosting confidence, mood and productivity.[3] What separates elite performers and individuals who achieve their lifelong goals from the rest is their ability to steer their inner monologue towards positive outcomes (and away from doubt). They believe they will succeed. But elite performers recognize that failing in an endeavour, in an attempt to grow or achieve, doesn't make you a failure. Failure is inevitable when chasing lofty goals; it's a necessary part of the journey. The best athletes fail all the time. Failing doesn't make *you* a failure, it's simply an opportunity for growth. True failure is when you're too afraid to try, or fear the opinions of others so much you won't even make the attempt.

Reboot Your Internal Monologue

Try repeating the following phrase every morning while you shower, or write it down on a Post-It note and stick it to your mirror:

> *I am willing.*
> *I embrace uncertainty.*
> *I am not my thoughts; I am my actions.*

Or create your own short phrases that relate to your values and goals, and repeat them every morning.

Mindfulness.

Mindfulness is focusing your attention on the process (and not the future outcome). In order to have a greater awareness of your thoughts, you need to build the skill of attention. Today, we live in a world with a wealth of information, but a poverty of attention. Mindfulness is the ability to place your full attention on what is happening right now, cutting through the 'busyness' noise of life like a hot knife through butter.

Staying Present

It's human nature to look ahead into the distance to see if you've reached your goal (like kids in the back of the car yelling, 'Are we there yet?'), but staying present is a key characteristic of high performers. It can feel like everyone else is hitting their goals and you ask yourself, why not me? For example, everyone can *seem* to be achieving rapid weight loss on social media (despite the reality being very different), which can amplify anxiety and sabotage your consistency. This leads to short-term thinking and a shot-gun approach to diet, exercise and lifestyle changes. If the latest popular diet doesn't work for you, you move on to another, looking for a quick fix. The truth is, no matter what diet you choose, there will always be roadblocks. Determining the right strategy to overcome them can be difficult and take a little time. The best predictor of success – in weight loss, nutrition or training – is compliance. Simply showing up every day, putting one foot in front of the other and committing to the process is the 'secret' to success. (And most clients fail to celebrate it.) But if you're constantly thinking about your future goal and why you're not achieving it, it will breed anxiety, which can derail consistency and your ability to focus on the process in the present moment.

Recent studies on mindfulness have revealed that it improves your coping response to stress and limits avoidance (a major win

Step 4 - Learn the Right Mindset Skills

Entire books are written on the subject, but I'll share a couple of techniques I've found useful and effective to get clients started.

Mindful Breathing

Taking a page from the Navy SEALs playbook, this exercise is called the 4-minute drill:

> Inhale for 4 seconds
> Exhale for 4 seconds
> Repeat for 4 minutes (And you're done!)

It's a great strategy to curb irritation, restlessness or anxiety when the pressure mounts (like heading into enemy territory!).

Mindfulness Immersion

If you're struggling to find time for mindfulness, insert *mindfulness immersion* into what you are already doing with your time.

Mindfulness immersion is the practice of using mundane tasks – like doing the dishes, the laundry or cleaning up around the house – to 'turn off' your thinking brain and shift your focus deeply into your household chores. (Let's face it, there is no shortage of those tasks in mid life!) Forget your deadlines and your to-do lists; dial all your attention into the task at hand.

Performing mundane tasks is a common theme in many spiritual practices. In Zen Buddhism, there is a saying: 'Before enlightenment, chop wood, carry water. After enlightenment, chop wood, carry water.' This underscores the notion that achieving your goal is not the endpoint and that even once you've achieved your goal, you'll still need to put the work in. Cultivating the skill of attention, via mindfulness, will serve you on your journey both to accomplishing your goals, as well as afterwards, for the more challenging hurdle of maintaining them.

when trying to resolve a weight-loss plateau or chronic health challenge), it improves emotional regulation, leading to better resilience, and it reduces symptoms of low mood and depression.[4] Do you ever feel anxious, irritated or easily annoyed? What about a persistent sensation of worry or anxiety? Does your mind often feel frenetic or overly critical towards yourself? Are your energy levels flat? Mindfulness has been shown to improve all of these areas (and then some). Mindfulness also helps to downshift an overactive nervous system, providing a feeling of relaxation that benefits memory and focus, blood pressure and heart rate, as well as a feeling of connectedness with others.[5]

Optimism

To achieve PEAK40 health and performance, optimism is essential. Optimism is intimately linked to motivation; optimistic

Imagine Your Best Self

New research has found that a daily, five-minute session of imagining your 'best self' can improve optimism. I use a variation of this exercise with weight-loss clients.

Imagine you've achieved your weight-loss goal and write down a detailed description of how you feel in your new body.

- What new emotions or sensations do you experience?
- What new identity do you take on?
- What new relationships have you built (or what old ones have you extinguished)?

Really lean into the exercise; clearly define how it looks and how it feels to be 'that person'. Have you imagined it? Once you have that picture clearly in your mind, ask yourself a question: how many of those attributes could you apply to yourself, today? Do you really have to wait until you've achieved 'success' on the scales to take on those feelings, behaviours and identity? Almost always, the answer is no.

The difference is the six inches between your ears. The difference is your mindset. Optimism helps to light the torch and extinguish the constant drip of negative thoughts and self-doubt.

people are more motivated, they exert more effort and they tend to have more social connections.[6] Optimism also bestows increased resilience to you for dealing with stressful life events – an important skill in the busy traffic of mid life.[7] Optimists are also more likely to believe a stressful event now can lead to a better and brighter future.[8] At the broadest level, optimism has protective properties for both mental and physical health, largely via its effects on health-promoting behaviours.[9] These are all crucial to successful behaviour change.

It was once thought that you were either an optimistic or pessimistic person. However, more recently scientists have uncovered that rather than being a hardwired personality trait, optimism is a skill that can be trained. The challenge is building optimism.

Become More by Being More, Not Doing More

The mindset skills of positive self-talk, the ability to maintain attention (aka mindfulness) and an optimistic outlook are the mortar that keep your values firmly in place, orienting you solidly towards your goals. Do you know your values? Do your behaviours align with those values? The challenge is battling through the cacophony and noise of daily life to find a quiet moment. You don't just need silence from the noise of the world, you need the space to uncover the silence within you. This was a revelation Erling Kagge experienced before he set out on his gruelling 50-day odyssey across Antarctica. But you don't need sub-zero temperatures to find silence; silence can be found anywhere and at any time. Don't wait for it to get quiet; create your own silence.

CHAPTER 13

Silence, Nature and Awe

'There is no path to happiness: happiness is the path.'
— GAUTAMA BUDDHA, philosopher

The sunset was spectacular. On a tiny, postage-stamp-size island in the archipelago of San Blas off the Atlantic coast of Panama, in the middle of what seems to be an endless ocean, I was completely alone – a voluntary castaway on a deserted island, in the middle of nowhere, surrounded by silence, easily the furthest I've ever been from another human being. The nature was awe-inspiring; I felt like I was at its mercy. I could see only the silhouette of other islands way off in the distance. My host Arnulfo, a local tribesman of the Kuna people, paddled in every morning with food (and small talk) for the day. I wasn't really stranded, nor completely isolated. But it felt like it. Arnulfo would stay for a few hours and when he left in his dugout canoe, I was alone again and swallowed up by the vastness of the blue water and the silence of the wind; awestruck by the power and beauty of nature.

Awe Ignites the Right Mindset

All of your thoughts are bathed in emotion. Building mindset skills allows you to direct those emotions and thoughts in a positive direction, so you can propel yourself to PEAK40 health and performance. The right mindset is a trainable skill and using strategies like optimism, mindfulness and self-talk, you can build a robust skillset to direct your thoughts. However, if you're struggling to kick-start the process, there is another way to ignite the journey. It's a very human emotion – feeling awestruck.

What Is Awe?

Awe isn't just a powerful emotion, it's a powerful *positive* emotion.[1] It's also been the subject of much research over the last half-decade. The scientific definition of awe is 'an intense emotional response to perceptually vast stimuli that dramatically transcend one's ordinary reference frame and provokes a need to adjust the current mental structures.'[2] A very granular way of saying an experience that re-opens your mind and shifts your mindset.

What creates awe? Scenes of natural beauty, like oceans, mountains, forests, animals in nature, spectacular sunrises and sunsets, incredible works of art or inspirational speeches, the collective exuberance of a stadium of cheering fans at a concert or sporting event, the birth of your child, or your religious or spiritual practices can all evoke the strong emotional response of awe. Awe includes feelings of wonder, amazement, elation, admiration and appreciation (and, of course, a little fear and anxiety in some circumstances, too!).[3]

Why Commit to Awe?

Even thinking about these types of events can take your mind in a different direction. Scientists are starting to uncover that your tendency to seek out 'awe moments' in your life is tied to some impressive cognitive changes. The more open you are to experiencing awe, the more transformational it can be to your mindset. The technical term is 'dispositional awe' and it represents your tendency, or likelihood, to experience awe.[4] For example, the experience of awe shifts your focus to the bigger picture (i.e. family, spirituality, happiness, etc).[5] The experience of awe diminishes the value you attach to excessive material goals.[6] The experience of awe can even give you a new perspective in your life.[7] That's incredibly powerful. (Particularly in mid life when happiness ebbs to a lifetime low.)

Committing to experiencing more awe in your life has been shown to:

- lower daily concerns
- reduce mundane desires
- diminish the emphasis on the individual self
- shift attention towards the needs of others
- encourage engagement in prosocial behaviours[8]

Awe transforms the way you think, away from self and towards the greater whole (which, coincidentally, is towards happiness).

I Don't Have Time for Awe!

If you can begin to find little moments of awe in your day, new research shows it increases your daily well-being (aka happiness). It's not only psychological, but physiological, as well. Awe is also a powerful signal and helps to turn down the inflammatory noise in the body. The more awe moments you experience, the lower your levels of inflammation.[9]

In a world where you seemingly have no time, awe has been shown to expand your perception of time.[10] In the same way that time can seem to stand still when doing squats or pull-ups, awe broadens our perception of time (without the discomfort!). In a world where rates of anxiety and depression are sky-rocketing, awe moments ignite people's love for life.[11] Don't have easy access to an ocean or forest? No problem, just being in a nature setting, like a local park, is enough to elicit awe and enhance well-being.[12]

How likely are you to experience or acknowledge awe moments in your day-to-day life? Weekly? Monthly? Only on vacation? (Pretty difficult in the daily grind of mid life, right?) Take a moment to reflect. They're actually happening all around you. Research from Amie Gordon, PhD, at the University of California at Berkeley, uncovered that awe moments are more common than you think in daily life, with study participants experiencing them on average every three days. So, where are all these effervescent awe moments hiding in your life? Here are a few evidence-based suggestions:

- stand under or gaze at tall trees
- reflect on travels or experiences in your past when you felt awestruck
- read poetry or song lyrics, focusing on the phrase or idea that connects with you
- connect with the main character of a story that creates a feeling of awe
- use social media to view awe-striking landscapes or binspiring speeches

Why does it matter? Awe saturates your mindset with a sense of meaning and fulfilment.[13] Brief experiences of awe also stimulate wonder and curiosity. Awe opens your mind to new possibilities, where 'something great' is just around the corner, and opens your mind to embrace new beliefs and behaviours.[14] All of this enhances your probability of experiencing positive meaning in your life.

Awe, Happiness and Life Meaning

We started off PEAK40 discussing happiness and how, in mid life, it may be at an all-time low. In science, terms must be defined in order to study them appropriately. Let's unpack happiness.

Happiness is labelled as subjective well-being, in the research, which is defined as your overall evaluation of your life.[15] This evaluation encompasses two main components: life satisfaction and subjective happiness.[16] What is life satisfaction? It's the analytical assessment of your life. As outlined in Chapter 1, financial success is strongly linked to life satisfaction. Subjective happiness, meanwhile, is the U-shaped curve described by Blanchflower; it's your overall assessment of whether you're happy or unhappy in your life. The key here is to highlight the difference between the rational side of happiness (i.e. life satisfaction) and the emotional side (i.e. subjective happiness). Cultivating dispositional awe is positively associated with both life satisfaction *and* subjective well-being.

Expert psychologists agree that having an overarching aim in one's life is an essential component for self-transcendence; the benevolence and universalism themes that connect us as humans.[17] The experience of awe is also in alignment with the concept of self-transcendence; overcoming the limits of your individual self (and its desires) and growing as a person throughout your life. When you experience awe, you're more likely to ponder the meaning of life, more likely to endorse more spiritual beliefs and more likely to reassess your life goals.[18] If you've lost your happiness compass, awe is your North Star.

Awe and Happiness: The Spark and the Torch

Inspiration is a central theme of awe.[19] Inspiration leads to motivation, motivation to discipline and discipline to habits. Only habits lead to automaticity; doing away with having to make a decision. This is where the greatest gains are made. You don't ask yourself 'if' you should get out of bed in the morning to exercise, you just do. You don't ask yourself 'if' you should have a high-protein snack in the afternoon, you just do. You don't ask yourself 'if' you should get to bed on time to feel rested the next day, you just do.

Step 4 – Kick-Start Your Path to Happiness

People who experience great subjective well-being, or happiness, tend to do the following:

- look for moments of awe in their day
- focus on what they have (not what they don't)
- have a few close friends
- compare themselves to themselves (not to others)

Taking a moment to appreciate what you have and to express gratitude for it is a powerful tool. However, just like sleep, it's the application of gratitude that's the challenge. Let's be honest, starting your day with a 15-minute journaling session when you've got kids at home is never going to happen. Never. Going. To. Happen. Instead, make it fit your lifestyle.

1. Every day (preferably in the morning), think of one thing you're grateful for in your life. Then say it out loud, 'I'm grateful for....' You can do it in the shower, in the car, or even muttered under your breath as you finally get the kids to school, whatever suits. But do it every day for a week. It might seem a little cheesy, but studies show this simple strategy can boost mood in a significant way. One thought of gratitude. (And while you're doing it, take one deep, full breath.) One thought of gratitude and one full breath. That's it. Commit to it.

2. Next, stop comparing yourself to others. Instead, compare yourself to *you* from last year, two years ago, or even five years ago. Pick a metric and compete against yourself; it's the only comparison that matters. What skills help to keep your mindset away from comparison? Positive self-talk, building optimism, establishing a personal philosophy and cultivating your ability to hold attention (to rein in the wandering mind) are all key skills to build a bulletproof mindset.

3. Help others. Today, in a world of constant distractions, time is the most precious thing you can give someone. Helping others doesn't just provide support for someone who needs it, it also provides massive fulfilment for those volunteering their time. It reminds you how fortunate you are and how grateful you should feel for what you have. It also improves wise reasoning, your ability to see the world from another person's point of view. In our modern, artificially intelligent world, wisdom will become the scarcest and most valuable commodity.

Closing Thoughts

Awe sparks the match, inspiration lights the fire and your mindset keeps the flames burning in the long run. You can only control your attitude, effort, actions and thoughts. That's it. How you view your situation, how you talk to yourself and how you envision your future shapes your subconscious. It's entirely in your control and you don't have to wait until you've lost weight, got a promotion or found someone special to ignite the process.

Awe and wonder are the engines of life. Look at your children (or a child) across the dinner table; you can see the curiosity in their eyes. The wonder and amazement at the end of each question. Questions, questions and more questions; they live in awe. Your head in mid life seems to get more filled with ambition than questions. Pause for a moment and give them your full attention. See the world through their eyes. Ask questions. It all starts with mindset.

Have You Heard the Parable of the Two Travellers and the Monk?

A traveller comes down the hill from the village in the mountain en route to the village in the valley. As he walks past a monk working in the field, he says, 'I'm on my way to the village in the valley, can you tell me what it's like?'

The monk stops what he is doing, looks up at the traveller and asks, 'Where have you come from?'

The traveller responds, 'I have come from the village in the mountains.'

'What was it like?' the monk asks.

'Terrible,' the man replies. 'Nobody spoke my language, I had to sleep in a barn, they fed me strange food and the weather was terrible.'

The monk responds, 'I think you'll find the village in the valley is much the same.'

A few hours later another traveller passes by, also coming from the hills and heading towards the valley below. The second traveller also spots the monk and asks, 'I'm on my way to the village in the valley, can you tell me what it's like?'

The monk stops what he is doing, looks up at the traveller and asks, 'Where have you come from?'

The second traveller replies, 'I have come from the village in the mountains.'

'What was it like?' enquires the monk.

'It was incredible,' exclaims the traveller. 'Nobody spoke my language so we communicated using hand and facial gestures. I slept in a barn under the stars for the first time in my life. I ate exotic new foods I had never tried. And the weather was cold, which made sitting by the fire such an amazing experience!'

'I see. I think you'll find the village in the valley is much the same,' responds the monk.

———

Mid life is demanding, stressful and relentless. It's also the greatest time to give, to love and to become. Life is 10 per cent what happens to you and 90 per cent how you respond. Acknowledge the awe-moments. Open up to optimism. And build the right habits. PEAK40 health and performance is just around the corner.

NOTES

Introduction: The Mid-Life U-Turn

1. 'Obesity and Overweight,' WHO Fact Sheets, World Health Organisation, accessed October 30, 2020, https://www.who.int/en/news-room/fact-sheets/detail /obesity-and-overweight; 'Preventing Noncommunicable Diseases,' WHO Activities, World Health Organisation, https://www.who.int/activities/preventing -noncommunicable-diseases.
2. Paul A. O'Keefe et al., 'Thinking beyond Boundaries: A Growth Theory of Interest Enhances Integrative Thinking that Bridges the Arts and Sciences,' *Organizational Behavior and Human Decision Processes* 162, no. 95 (January 2021): 95–108, https://doi.org/10.1016/j.obhdp.2020.10.007.
3. Chip Heath and Dan Heath, *Switch* (New York: Random House Business, 2011).

Chapter 1: The Mid-Life Happiness Curve

1. David Blanchflower, 'Is Happiness U-shaped Everywhere? Age and Subjective Well-being in 132 Countries,' National Bureau of Economic Research (January 2020), https://www.nber.org/papers/w26641.
2. Sonja Lyubomirsky, 'Hedonic Adaptation to Positive and Negative Experiences,' in *The Oxford Handbook of Stress, Health, and Coping* (January 2012), https://doi.org /10.1093/oxfordhb/9780195375343.013.0011.
3. William G. Iacono and Matt McGue, 'Minnesota Twin Family Study,' *Twin Research* 5, no. 5 (October 2002): 482–7, https://doi.org/10.1375/136905202320906327.
4. Dr Peter Jensen, 'Sport Psychology, Energy Management & the Champion's Mindset,' interview by Dr Marc Bubbs, *The Performance Nutrition Podcast,* September 13, 2018, https://soundcloud.com/drbubbs/s2e35-sport-psychology-energy -management-the-champions-mindset-dr-peter-jensen.
5. F. P. Cappuccio et al., 'Sleep Duration and All-Cause Mortality: A Systematic Review and Meta-analysis of Prospective Studies,' *Sleep* 33, no. 5 (2010), https:// doi.org/10.1111/j.1365-2869.2008.00732.x.
6. Jacob A. Nota and Meredith E. Coles, 'Duration and Timing of Sleep Are Associated with Repetitive Negative Thinking,' *Cognitive Therapy and Research* 39, no. 2 (April 2015): 253–61, https://doi.org/10.1007/s10608-014-9651-7.
7. J. C. Felger and F. E. Lotrich, 'Inflammatory Cytokines in Depression: Neurobiological Mechanisms and Therapeutic Implications,' *Neuroscience* 246 (2013), https://doi.org/10.1016/j.neuroscience.2013.04.060.
8. Antti-Jussi Pyykkönen et al., 'Depressive Symptoms, Antidepressant Medication Use, and Insulin Resistance: The PPP-Botnia Study,' *Diabetes Care* 34, no. 12 (December 2011): 2545–7, https://doi.org/10.2337/dc11-0107.

9. Markku Timonen et al., 'Insulin Resistance and Depressive Symptoms in Young Adult Males: Findings from Finnish Military Conscripts,' *Psychosomatic Medicine* 69, no. 8 (October 2007): 723–8, https://doi.org/10.1097/psy.0b013e318157ad2e.

10. The Emerging Risk Factors Collaboration, 'Diabetes Mellitus, Fasting Glucose, and Risk of Cause-Specific Death,' *New England Journal of Medicine* 364, no. 9 (March 2011): 829–41, https://doi.org/10.1056/nejmoa1008862.

Chapter 2: Super Bowl or Heart Attack?

1. Emelia J. Benjamin et al., 'Heart Disease and Stroke Statistics–2018 Update: A Report from the American Heart Association,' *Circulation* 137, no.12 (January 2018): e67–492, https://doi.org/10.1161/CIR.0000000000000558.

2. Sébastien Lacroix et al., 'Contemporary Issues Regarding Nutrition in Cardiovascular Rehabilitation,' *Annals of Physical Rehabilitation Medicine* 60, no. 1 (January 2017): 36–42, https://doi.org/10.1016/j.rehab.2016.07.262; Sukriti Sukriti et al., 'Mechanisms Regulating Endothelial Permeability,' *Pulmonary Circulation* 4, no. 4 (December 2014): 535–551, https://doi.org/10.1086/677356; Lisa K. Jennings, 'Mechanisms of Platelet Activation: Need for New Strategies to Protect Against Platelet-Mediated Atherothrombosis,' *Journal of Thrombosis and Haemostasis* 102, no. 2 (2009): 248–57, https://doi.org/10.1160/TH09-03-0192; Renu Virmani et al., 'Recent Highlights of ATVB: Calcification,' *Arteriosclerosis, Thrombosis, and Vascular Biology* 34, no. 7 (May 2014): 1329–32, https://doi.org/10.1161/ATVBAHA.114.304000.

3. Rik P. Bogers et al., 'Association of Overweight with Increased Risk of Coronary Heart Disease Partly Independent of Blood Pressure and Cholesterol Levels: A Meta-analysis of 21 Cohort Studies Including More Than 300,000 Persons,' *Archives of Internal Medicine* 167, no. 16 (2007): 1720–28, https://doi.org/10.1001/archinte.167.16.1720.

4. Andrew M. Tucker et al., 'Prevalence of Cardiovascular Disease Risk Factors among National Football League Players,' *JAMA* 301, no. 20 (2009): 2111–9, https://doi.org/10.1001/jama.2009.716.

5. S. Baron and R. Rinsky, 'Health Hazard Evaluation Report: HETA – 88 – 085, National Football League Players Mortality Study,' *National Institute for Occupational Safety and Health* (January 1994): 1–13, https://www.cdc.gov/niosh/hhe/reports/pdfs/1988-0085-letter.pdf.

6. Sherry L. Baron et al., 'Body Mass Index, Playing Position, Race, and the Cardiovascular Mortality of Retired Professional Football Players,' *The American Journal of Cardiology* 109, no. 6 (January 2012), https://doi.org/10.1016/j.amjcard.2011.10.050.

7. J. V. Bjørnholt et al., 'Fasting Blood Glucose: An Underestimated Risk Factor for Cardiovascular Death. Results from a 22-year Follow-up of Healthy Nondiabetic Men," *Diabetes Care* 22, no. 1 (January 1999): 45–9, https://doi.org/10.2337/diacare.22.1.45.

8. J. H. Fuller et al., 'Mortality from Coronary Heart Disease and Stroke in Relation to Degree of Glycaemia: The Whitehall Study,' *British Medical Journal (Clinical Research Edition)* 287, no. 867 (September 1983), https://doi.org/10.1136/bmj.287.6396.867.

9. Elizabeth Barrett-Connor et al., 'Is Borderline Fasting Hyperglycemia a Risk Factor for Cardiovascular Death?' *Journal of Chronic Diseases* 37, no. 9–10 (1984): 773–9, https://doi.org/10.1016/0021-9681(84)90046-8.

10. J. Pérez-Jiménez et al., 'Identification of the 100 Richest Dietary Sources of Polyphenols: An Application of the Phenol-Explorer Database,' *European Journal of Clinical Nutrition* 64, Supplement 3 (November 2010), https://doi.org/10.1038/ejcn.2010.221.

11. Sohaib Haseeb et al., 'Wine and Cardiovascular Health: A Comprehensive Review,' *Circulation* 136, no. 15 (October 2017): 1434–48, https://doi.org/10.1161/CIRCULATIONAHA.117.030387; Sohaib Haseeb et al., 'What's in Wine? A Clinician's Perspective,' *Trends in Cardiovascular Medicine* 29, no.2 (February 2019): 97–106, https://doi.org/10.1016/j.tcm.2018.06.010.

12. Kim Sutton-Tyrell et al., 'Study of Women's Health Across the Nation (SWAN), 2003-2005: Visit 07 Dataset,' *Nutr. Aging* 2, no. 2-3 (November 2018), https://doi.org/10.3886/ICPSR31901.v2.

13. Simona Costano et al., 'Wine, Beer or Spirit Drinking in Relation to Fatal and Nonfatal Cardiovascular Events: A Meta-analysis,' *European Journal of Epidemiology* 26, no. 11 (November 2011): 833–50, https://doi.org/10.1007/s10654-011-9631-0.

14. S. G. Wannamethee and A. G. Shaper, 'Type of Alcoholic Drink and Risk of Major Coronary Heart Disease Events and All-cause Mortality,' *American Journal of Public Health* 89, no. 5 (May 1999), https://doi.org/10.2105/ajph.89.5.685.

15. Ben Crair and Andrew Keh, 'German Olympians Drink a Lot of (Nonalcoholic) Beer, and Win a Lot of Gold Medals,' *New York Times,* February 19, 2018, https://www.nytimes.com/2018/02/19/sports/olympics/germany-olympics-beer.html.

16. G. Chiva-Blanch et al., 'Effects of Alcohol and Polyphenols from Beer on Atherosclerotic Biomarkers in High Cardiovascular Risk Men: A Randomized Feeding Trial,' *Nutrition, Metabolism & Cardiovascular Disease* 25, no. 1 (January 2015): 36–45, https://doi.org/10.1016/j.numecd.2014.07.008.

17. Ben Bikman, 'Why We Get Sick – Hyperinsulinemia & Chronic Disease,' interview by Dr Marc Bubbs, *Performance Nutrition Podcast,* November 24, 2020, https://www.athleteevolution.org/season-4-performance-nutrition-podcast/s4e18-why-we-get-sick-hyper-insulinemia-amp-chronic-disease-w-dr-ben-bikman-phd.

18. Rosa Casas et al., 'Nutrition and Cardiovascular Health,' *International Journal of Molecular Science* 19, no. 12 (November 2018): 3988, https://doi.org/10.3390/ijms19123988; Dariush Mozaffarian, 'Dietary and Policy Priorities for Cardiovascular Disease, Diabetes, and Obesity: A Comprehensive Review,' *Circulation* 133, no. 2 (January 2016): 187–225, https://doi.org/10.1161/CIRCULATIONAHA.115.018585; Dariush Mozaffarian and David Ludwig, 'Dietary Guidelines in the 21st Century – a Time for Food,' *JAMA* 304, no. 6 (August 2010): 681–2, https://doi.org/10.1001/jama.2010.1116; Renate Micha et al., 'Association Between Dietary Factors and Mortality from Heart Disease, Stroke, and Type 2 Diabetes in the United States,' *JAMA* 317, no.9 (March 2017): 912–24, https://doi.org/10.1001/jama.2017.0947.

Chapter 3: The Blood-Sugar Rollercoaster

1. Yan Zheng et al., 'Associations of Weight Gain from Early to Middle Adulthood with Major Health Outcomes Later in Life,' *JAMA* 318, no. 3 (July 2017): 255–69, https://doi.org/10.1001/jama.2017.7092.

2. 'Obesity and Overweight,' WHO Fact Sheets, World Health Organization, accessed October 2020, http://www.who.int/mediacentre/factsheets/fs311/en/; Adela Hruby et al., 'Determinants and Consequences of Obesity,' *American Journal of Public Health* 106, no. 9 (September 2016), https://doi.org/10.2105/AJPH .2016.303326.

3. Earl S. Ford et al., 'Prevalence of the Metabolic Syndrome among US Adults: Findings from the Third National Health and Nutrition Examination Survey,' *JAMA* 287, no. 3 (January 2002): 356–9, https://doi.org/10.1001/jama.287.3.356.

4. J. V. Bjørnholt et al., 'Fasting Blood Glucose: An Underestimated Risk Factor for Cardiovascular Death. Results from a 22-year Follow-up of Healthy Nondiabetic Men," *Diabetes Care* 22, no. 1 (January 1999): 45–9, https://doi.org/10.2337/diacare.22.1.45.

5. Sang-Wook Yi et al., 'Association Between Fasting Glucose and All-Cause Mortality According to Sex and Age: A Prospective Cohort Study," *Scientific Reports* 7, no. 8194 (August 2017), https://doi.org/10.1038/s41598-017-08498-6.

6. Andy Menke et al., 'Prevalence of and Trends in Diabetes among Adults in the United States, 1988–2012,' *JAMA* 314, no. 10 (September 2015): 1021–9, https:// doi.org/10.1001/jama.2015.10029; Earl S. Ford et al., 'Prevalence of the Metabolic Syndrome Among US Adults: Findings from the Third National Health and Nutrition Examination Survey,' *JAMA* 287, no. 3 (January 2002): 356–9, https:// doi.org/10.1001/jama.287.3.356; J. H. Fuller et al., 'Mortality from Coronary Heart Disease and Stroke in Relation to Degree of Glycaemia: The Whitehall Study,' *British Medical Journal (Clinical Research Edition)* 287, no. 6396 (September 1983), https://doi.org/10.1136/bmj.287.6396.867.

7. David Stuckler et al., 'Manufacturing Epidemics: The Role of Global Producers in Increased Consumption of Unhealthy Commodities Including Processed Foods, Alcohol, and Tobacco,' *PLoS Med* 9, no. 6 (June 2012), https://doi.org/10.1371 /journal.pmed.1001235; C. A. Monteiro et al., 'Ultra-processed Products Are Becoming Dominant in the Global Food System,' *Obesity Reviews* 14, no. S2 (September 2013), https://doi.org/10.1111/obr.12107.

8. Euridice Martínez Steele et al., 'Ultra-processed Foods, Protein Leverage and Energy Intake in the USA," *Public Health Nutrition* 21, no. 1 (January 2018): 114–24, https://doi.org/10.1017/S1368980017001574; Laura Schnabel et al., 'Association Between Ultraprocessed Food Consumption and Risk of Mortality Among Middle-Aged Adults in France,' *JAMA Internal Med.* 179, no. 4 (February 2019): 490–8, https://doi.org/10.1001/jamainternmed.2018.7289; Thibault Fiolet et al., 'Consumption of Ultra-processed Foods and Cancer Risk: Results from NutriNet-Santé Prospective Cohort," *BMJ* 360, no. 322 (February 2018), https://doi.org/10.1136/bmj.k322.

9. Danilo Cosme Klein Gomes et al., 'Trends in Obesity Prevalence among Brazilian Adults from 2002 to 2013 by Educational Level,' *BMC Public Health* 19, no. 965 (July 2019), https://doi.org/10.1186/s12889-019-7289-9.

10. Carlos Augusto Monteiro et al., 'The UN Decade of Nutrition, the NOVA Food Classification and the Trouble with Ultra-processing,' *Public Health Nutrition* 21, no. 1 (January 2018): 5–17, https://doi.org/10.1017/S1368980017000234.

11. Michael J. Gibney et al., 'Ultra-processed Foods in Human Health: A Critical Appraisal,' *The American Journal of Clinical Nutrition* 106, no. 3 (September 2017): 717–24, https://doi.org/10.3945/ajcn.117.160440.

12. Anastassia Gorvitovskaia et al., 'Interpreting *Prevotella* and *Bacteroides* as Biomarkers of Diet and Lifestyle,' *Microbiome* 4, no. 15 (April 2016), https://doi.org/10.1186/s40168-016-0160-7.

13. Jennifer M. Poti et al., 'Ultra-processed Food Intake and Obesity: What Really Matters for Health – Processing or Nutrient Content?' *Current Obesity Reports* 6, no. 4 (October 2017): 420–31, https://doi.org/10.1007/s13679-017-0285-4.

14. Jennifer M. Poti et al., 'Is the Degree of Food Processing and Convenience Linked with the Nutritional Quality of Foods Purchased by US Households?' *The American Journal of Clinical Nutrition* 101, no. 6 (June 2015): 1251–62, https://doi.org/10.3945/ajcn.114.100925.

15. Erica M. Schulte et al., 'Which Foods May Be Addictive? The Roles of Processing, Fat Content, and Glycemic Load,' *PLoS ONE* 10, no. 2 (February 2015), https://doi.org/10.1371/journal.pone.0117959.

16. Kevin D. Hall et al., 'Ultra-processed Diets Cause Excess Calorie Intake and Weight Gain: An Inpatient Randomized Controlled Trial of *Ad Libitum* Food Intake,' *Cell Metabolism* 30, no. 1 (May 2019): 67–77, https://doi.org/10.1016/j.cmet.2019.05.008.

17. Emma J. Stinson et al., 'High Fat and Sugar Consumption During *Ad Libitum* Intake Predicts Weight Gain,' *Obesity* 26, no. 4 (March 2018), https://doi.org/10.1002/oby.22124.

18. Amy A. Gorin et al., 'Randomized Controlled Trial Examining the Ripple Effect of a Nationally Available Weight Management Program on Untreated Spouses,' *Obesity* 26, no. 3 (February 2018), https://doi.org/10.1002/oby.22098.

19. Bernard Srour et al., 'Ultraprocessed Food Consumption and Risk of Type 2 Diabetes among Participants of the NutriNet-Santé Prospective Cohort,' *JAMA Internal Medicine* 180, no. 2 (December 2019): 283-91, https://doi.org/10.1001/jamainternmed.2019.5942.

Chapter 4: Master Your Morning

1. James A. Betts et al., 'The Causal Role of Breakfast in Energy Balance and Health: a Randomized Controlled Trial in Lean Adults,' *The American Journal of Clinical Nutrition* 100, no. 2 (August 2014): 539–47, https://doi.org/10.3945/ajcn.114.083402.

2. Charles Spence, 'Breakfast: The Most Important Meal of the Day?,' *International Journal of Gastronomy and Food Science* 8 (July 2017): 1–6, https://doi.org/10.1016/j.ijgfs.2017.01.003.

3. Emily J. Dhurandhar et al., 'The Effectiveness of Breakfast Recommendations on Weight Loss: A Randomized Controlled Trial,' *The American Journal of Clinical Nutrition* 100, no.2 (August 2014): 507–13, https://doi.org/10.3945/ajcn.114.089573.

4. Katherine Sievert et al., 'Effect of Breakfast on Weight and Energy Intake: Systematic Review and Meta-analysis of Randomised Controlled Trials," *BMJ* 364, no. 142 (January 2019), https://doi.org/10.1136/bmj.l42.

5. Tomoya Mita et al., 'Breakfast Skipping Is Associated with Persistently Increased Arterial Stiffness in Patients with Type 2 Diabetes,' *BMJ Open Diabetes Research and Care* 8, no. 1 (February 2020), https://doi.org/10.1136/bmjdrc-2019-001162.

6. Amber A.W.A. van der Heijden et al., 'A Prospective Study of Breakfast Consumption and Weight Gain among U.S. Men,' *Obesity* 15, no. 10 (September 2012), https://doi.org/10.1038/oby.2007.292.

7. Rania A. Mekary et al., 'Eating Patterns and Type 2 Diabetes Risk in Men: Breakfast Omission, Eating Frequency, and Snacking,' *The American Journal of Clinical Nutrition* 95, no. 5 (May 2012): 1182–9, https://doi.org/10.3945/ajcn.111.028209; Irina Uzhova et al., 'The Importance of Breakfast in Atherosclerosis Disease: Insights from the PESA Study,' *Journal of the American College of Cardiology* 70, no. 15 (October 2017): 1833–42, https://doi.org/10.1016/j.jacc.2017.08.027.

8. Leah Cahill et al., 'Prospective Study of Breakfast Eating and Incident Coronary Heart Disease in a Cohort of Male US Health Professionals,' Circulation 128, no. 4 (July 2013): 337–343, https://doi.org/10.1161/CIRCULATIONAHA.113.001474; Kenneth Anujuo et al., 'Relationship between Sleep Duration and Artierla Stifness in Multi-ethnic Population: The HELIUS Study,' *Chronbiol International Journal of Public Health* 33, no. 5 (April 2016): 543–552, https://doi.org/10.3109/07420528.2016.1158721.

9. Leah Cahill et al., 'Prospective Study of Breakfast Eating and Incident Coronary Heart Disease in a Cohort of Male US Health Professionals,' *Circulation* 128, no. 4 (July 2013): 337–43, https://doi.org/10.1161/CIRCULATIONAHA.113.001474; Yasuhiko Kubota et al., 'Association of Breakfast Intake with Incident Stroke and Coronary Heart Disease: The Japan Public Health Center-Based Study,' *Stroke* 47, no. 2 (January 2016): 477–81, https://doi.org/10.1161/STROKEAHA.115.011350; Shuang Rong et al., 'Association of Skipping Breakfast with Cardiovascular and All-Cause Mortality,' *Journal of the American College of Cardiology* 73, no. 16 (April 2019): 2025–32, https://doi.org/10.1016/j.jacc.2019.01.065.

10. Jihui Zhang et al., 'Relationship of Sleep Quantity and Quality with 24-Hour Urinary Catecholamines and Salivary Awakening Cortisol in Healthy Middle-Aged Adults,' *Sleep* 34, no. 2 (February 2011): 225–33, https://doi.org/10.1093/sleep/34.2.225.

11. Daniela Jakubowicz et al., 'Fasting until Noon Triggers Increased Postprandial Hyperglycemia and Impaired Insulin Response after Lunch and Dinner in

Individuals with Type 2 Diabetes: A Randomized Clinical Trial,' *Diabetes Care* 38, no. 10 (October 2015), https://doi.org/10.2337/dc15-0761.

12. Javier T. Gonzalez et al., 'Molecular Adaptations of Adipose Tissue to 6 Weeks of Morning Fasting vs. Daily Breakfast Consumption in Lean and Obese Adults,' *The Journal of Physiology* 596, no. 4 (November 2017), https://doi.org/10.1113/JP275113.

13. James A. Betts et al., 'Is Breakfast the Most Important Meal of the Day?,' *Proceedings of the Nutrition Society* 75, no. 4 (June 2016), https://doi.org/10.1017/S0029665116000318; Enhad A. Chowdhury et al., 'The Causal Role of Breakfast in Energy Balance and Health: A Randomized Controlled Trial in Obese Adults,' *The American Journal of Clinical Nutrition* 103, no. 3 (March 2016): 747–56, https://doi.org/10.3945/ajcn.115.122044.

14. R. Edinburgh et al., 'Skipping Breakfast Before Exercise Creates a More Negative 24-hour Energy Balance: A Randomized Controlled Trial in Healthy Physically Active Young Men,' *The Journal of Nutrition* 149, no. 8 (August 2019): 1326–34, https://doi.org/10.1093/jn/nxz018.

15. Emma J. Stinson et al., 'High Fat and Sugar Consumption During *Ad Libitum* Intake Predicts Weight Gain,' *Obesity* 26, no. 4 (March 2018), https://doi.org/10.1002/oby.22124.

16. D. Benton et al., 'The Influence of Breakfast and a Snack on Psychological Functioning,' *Physiology & Behavior* 74, no. 4–5 (November 2001), https://doi.org/10.1016/s0031-9384(01)00601-1.

Chapter 5: Own Your Night

1. Frank Scheer et al., 'Adverse Metabolic and Cardiovascular Consequences of Circadian Misalignment,' *Proceedings of the National Academy of Sciences of the United States of America* 106, no. 11 (March 2009): 4453–8, https://doi.org/10.1073/pnas.0808180106; J. Cleator et al., 'Night Eating Syndrome: Implications for Severe Obesity,' *Nutrition & Diabetes* 2, no. 9 (July 2012), https://doi.org/10.1038/nutd.2012.16; Daniela Jakubowicz et al., 'High Caloric Intake at Breakfast vs. Dinner Differentially Influences Weight Loss of Overweight and Obese Women,' *Obesity* 21, no. 12 (March 2013), https://doi.org/10.1002/oby.20460.

2. Andrew W. McHill et al., 'Later Circadian Timing of Food Intake Is Associated with Increased Body Fat,' *The American Journal of Clinical Nutrition* 106, no. 5 (November 2017): 1213–9, https://doi.org/10.3945/ajcn.117.161588.

3. Luciana Antunes et al., 'Obesity and Shift Work: Chronobiological Aspects,' *Nutrition Research Reviews* 23, no. 1(2010), https://doi:10.1017/S0954422410000016.

4. Judith Baird, 'Evening Eating Linked to Higher Total Caloric Intake, Lower Diet Quality,' *ECOICO* (2020), presented September 1–4, abstract 1065, LBA-056.

5. Alessa Nas et al., 'Impact of Breakfast Skipping Compared with Dinner Skipping on Regulation of Energy Balance and Metabolic Risk,' *The American Journal of Clinical Nutrition* 105, no. 6 (June 2017): 1351–61, https://doi.org/10.3945/ajcn.116.151332.

6. R. I. Versteeg et al., 'Serotonin, a Possible Intermediate between Disturbed Circadian Rhythms and Metabolic Disease,' *Neuroscience* 301 (August 2015): 155–67, https://doi.org/10.1016/j.neuroscience.2015.05.067; Andries Kalsbeek et al., 'Circadian Control of Glucose Metabolism,' *Molecular Metabolism* 3, no. 4 (July 2014): 372–83, https://doi.org/10.1016/j.molmet.2014.03.002.

7. Martin Brandhagen et al., 'Alcohol and Macronutrient Intake Patterns Are Related to General and Central Adiposity,' *European Journal of Clinical Nutrition* 66, no. 3 (2012), https://10.1038/ejcn.2011.189.

8. Leah E. Cahill et al., 'Prospective Study of Breakfast Eating and Incident Coronary Heart Disease in a Cohort of Male US Health Professionals,' *Circulation* 128, no. 4 (July 2013): 337–43, https://doi.org/10.1161/CIRCULATIONAHA.113.001474.

9. Junko Yoshida et al., 'Association of Night Eating Habits with Metabolic Syndrome and Its Components: A Longitudinal Study,' *BMC Public Health* 18, no. 1366 (2018), https://doi.org/10.1186/s12889-018-6262-3.

10. Shuang Rong et al., 'Association of Skipping Breakfast with Cardiovascular and All-Cause Mortality,' *Journal of the American College of Cardiology* 73, no. 16 (April 2019): 2025–32, https://doi.org/10.1016/j.jacc.2019.01.065; Suzana Almoosawi et al., 'Chrono-nutrition: A Review of Current Evidence from Observational Studies on Global Trends in Time-of-Day of Energy Intake and Its Association with Obesity,' *Proceedings of the Nutrition Society* 75, no. 4 (2016), https://doi:10.1017/S0029665116000306.

11. Frank A. J. L. Scheer et al., 'Adverse Metabolic and Cardiovascular Consequences of Circadian Misalignment,' *PNAS* 106, no. 11 (March 2009): 4453–8, https://doi.org/10.1073/pnas.0808180106; Marie-Pierre St-Onge et al., 'Meal Timing and Frequency: Implications for Cardiovascular Disease Prevention: A Scientific Statement from the American Heart Association,' *Circulation* 135, no. 9 (January 2017), https://doi.org/10.1161/CIR.0000000000000476.

12. Nirinjini Naidoo et al., 'Aging and Sleep Deprivation Induce the Unfolded Protein Response in the Pancreas: Implications for Metabolism,' *Aging Cell* 13, no. 1 (September 2013), https://doi.org/10.1111/acel.12158; Valeriy A. Poroyko et al., 'Chronic Sleep Disruption Alters Gut Microbiota, Induces Systemic and Adipose Tissue Inflammation and Insulin Resistance in Mice,' *Scientific Reports* 6, no. 35405 (October 2016), https://doi.org/10.1038/srep35405.

Chapter 6: Set Your Protein

1. Penny Kris-Etherton, 'Monounsaturated Fatty Acids and Risk of Cardiovascular Disease,' *Circulation* 100, no. 11 (September 1999): 1253–8, https://doi.org/10.1161/01.CIR.100.11.1253.

2. 'Scientific Report of the 2015 Dietary Guidelines Advisory Committee: Advisory Report to the Secretary of Health and Human Services and the Secretary of Agriculture (2015),' Dietary Guidelines Advisory Committee, accessed June 14, 2019, https://health.gov/dietaryguidelines/2015-scientific-report/.

3. Jose Antonio et al., 'A High Protein Diet Has No Harmful Effects: A One-Year Crossover Study in Resistance-Trained Males,' *Journal of Nutrition and Metabolism* 2016, no. 9104791 (October 2016), https://doi.org/10.1155/2016/9104792.

4. Professor Stuart Phillips, 'Dietary Supplements & the High Performance Athlete,' interview by Dr Marc Bubbs, *Performance Nutrition Podcast,* April 26, 2018, https://drbubbs.com/season-2-podcast-episodes/2018/4/s2-episode-17-dietary -supplements-the-high-performance-athlete-w-dr-stu-phillips-phd.

5. Renata Micha et al., 'Red and Processed Meat Consumption and Risk of Incident Coronary Heart Disease, Stroke, and Diabetes Mellitus: A Systematic Review and Meta-analysis,' *Circulation* 121, no. 21 (May 2010): 2271–83, https://doi.org /10.1161/CIRCULATIONAHA.109.924977.

6. Dena Zeraatkar et al., 'Effect of Lower Versus Higher Red Meat Intake on Cardio-metabolic and Cancer Outcomes: A Systematic Review of Randomized Trials,' *Annals of Internal Medicine* 171, no. 10 (November 2019): 721–31, https://doi.org /10.7326/M19-0622.

7. Lauren E. O'Connor et al., 'Total Red Meat Intake of ≥0.5 Servings/d Does Not Negatively Influence Cardiovascular Disease Risk Factors: A Systemically Searched Meta-analysis of Randomized Controlled Trials,' *The American Journal of Clinical Nutrition* 105, no.1 (January 2017): 57–69, https://doi.org/10.3945 /ajcn.116.142521.

8. Helena Sandoval-Insausti et al., 'Macronutrients Intake and Incident Frailty in Older Adults: A Prospective Cohort Study,' *The Journals of Gerontology: Series A* 71, no. 10 (October 2016): 1329–34, https://doi.org/10.1093/gerona/glw033.

9. Yue Wang et al., 'Higher Egg Consumption Associated with Increased Risk of Diabetes in Chinese Adults – China Health and Nutrition Survey,' *British Journal of Nutrition* 1–8 (October 2020), https://doi.org/10.1017/S0007114520003955.

10. Mahshid Dehghan et al., 'Association of Egg Intake with Blood Lipids, Cardiovascular Disease, and Mortality in 177,000 People in 50 Countries,' *The American Journal of Clinical Nutrition* 111 , mo. 4 (April 2020): 795–803, https:// doi.org/10.1093/ajcn/nqz348.

11. Nancy R. Rodriguez, 'Introduction to Protein Summit 2.0: Continued Explora-tion of the Impact of High-Quality Protein on Optimal Health,' *The American Journal of Clinical Nutrition* 101, no. 6 (June 2015): 1317S–1319S, https://doi .org/10.3945/ajcn.114.083980; Mercedes Sotos-Prieto et al., 'Association of Changes in Diet Quality with Total and Cause-Specific Mortality,' *The New England Journal of Medicine* 377, (July 2017): 143–53, https://doi.org/10.1056 /NEJMoa1613502.

12. '2015–2020 Dietary Guidelines for Americans 8th ed. (2015),' U.S. Department of Health and Human Services, U.S. Department of Agriculture, accessed October 19, 2019, http://health.gov/dietaryguidelines/2015/guidelines/.

13. Steven H. Zeisel and Kerry-Ann Da Costa, 'Choline: An Essential Nutrient for Public Health,' *Nutrition Reviews* 67, no. 11 (November 2009): 615–23, https://

doi.org/10.1111/j.1753-4887.2009.00246.x; Gilbert S. Omenn et al., 'Effects of a Combination of Beta Carotene and Vitamin A on Lung Cancer and Cardiovascular Disease,' *The New England Journal of Medicine* 334, no. 18 (May 1996): 1150–5, https://doi.org/10.1056/NEJM199605023341802; Connie M. Weaver, 'Potassium and Health,' *Advances in Nutrition* 4, no. 3 (May 2013): 368S–377S, https://doi.org/10.3945/an.112.003533; Jeroen H. F. de Baaij et al., 'Magnesium in Man: Implications for Health and Disease,' *Physiological Reviews* 95, no. 1 (January 2015), https://doi.org/10.1152/physrev.00012.2014; Henry C. Lukaski, 'Vitamin and Mineral Status: Effects on Physical Performance,' *Nutrition* 20, no. 7-8 (July–August 2004): 632–44, https://doi.org/10.1016/j.nut.2004.04.001; James P. McClung and Erin Gaffney-Stomberg, 'Optimizing Performance, Health, and Well-Being: Nutritional Factors,' *Military Medicine* 181, no. supp 1 (January 2016): 86–91, https://doi.org/10.7205/milmed-d-15-00202.

14. Carol E. O'Neil et al., 'Food Sources of Energy and Nutrients among Adults in the US: NHANES 2003–2006,' *Nutrients* 4, no. 12 (December 2012): 2097–120, https://doi.org/10.3390/nu4122097.

15. Jess A. Gwynn et al., 'Higher Protein Density Diets Are Associated with Greater Diet Quality and Micronutrient Intake in Healthy Young Adults,' *Frontiers in Nutrition* 6, no. 59 (May 2019), https://doi.org/10.3389/fnut.2019.00059; Peter J. Huth et al., 'Major Food Sources of Calories, Added Sugars, and Saturated Fat and Their Contribution to Essential Nutrient Intakes in the U.S. Diet: Data from the National Health,' *Nutrition Journal* 12, no. 116 (August 2013), https://doi.org/10.1186/1475-2891-12-116.

16. Jose Antonio et al., 'The Effects of Consuming a High Protein Diet (4.4 g/kg/d) on Body Composition in Resistance-Trained Individuals,' *Journal of the International Society of Sports Nutrition* 11, no. 19 (May 2014): https://doi.org/10.1186/1550-2783-11-19.

17. Daniel A. Traylor, Stefan H. M. Gorissen, and Stuart M. Phillips, 'Perspective: Protein Requirements and Optimal Intakes in Aging: Are We Ready to Recommend More Than the Recommended Daily Allowance?,' *Advances in Nutrition* 9, no. 3 (May 2018): 171–82, https://doi.org/10.1093/advances/nmy003.

18. Robert W. Morton et al., 'A Systematic Review, Meta-analysis and Meta-regression of the Effect of Protein Supplementation on Resistance Training-Induced Gains in Muscle Mass and Strength in Healthy Adults,' *British Journal of Sports Medicine* 5, no. 6 (2017), https://doi.org/10.1136/bjsports-2017-097608.

19. Ralf Jäger et al., 'International Society of Sports Nutrition Position Stand: Protein and Exercise,' *Journal of the International Society of Sports Nutrition* 14, no. 20 (June 2017), https://doi.org/10.1186/s12970-017-0177-8.

20. Eric R. Helms, Alan A. Aragon, and Peter J. Fitschen, 'Evidence-Based Recommendations for Natural Bodybuilding Contest Preparation: Nutrition and Supplementation,' *Journal of the International Society of Sports Nutrition* 11, no. 20 (May 2014), https://doi.org/10.1186/1550-2783-11-20.

21. Jess A. Gwin et al., 'Higher Protein Density Diets Are Associated with Greater Diet Quality and Micronutrient Intake in Healthy Young Adults,' *Frontiers in Nutrition* 6, no. 59 (May 2019), https://doi.org/10.3389/fnut.2019.00059.

Chapter 7: Turn The Dial on Carbs

1. An Pan et al., 'Diet and Cardiovascular Disease: Advances and Challenges in Population-Based Studies,' *Cell Metabolism* 27, no. 3 (March 2018): 489–96, https://doi.org/10.1016/j.cmet.2018.02.017.

2. Kazumasa Yamagishi et al., 'Plasma Fatty Acid Composition and Incident Heart Failure in Middle-aged Adults: The Atherosclerosis Risk in Communities (ARIC) Study,' *American Heart Journal* 156, no. 5 (November 2008): 965–74, https://doi.org/10.1016/j.ahj.2008.06.017; Eva Warensjö et al., 'Markers of Dietary Fat Quality and Fatty Acid Desaturation as Predictors of Total and Cardiovascular Mortality: A Population-Based Prospective Study,' *The American Journal of Clinical Nutrition* 88, no. 1 (July 2008): 203–9, https://doi.org/10.1093/ajcn/88.1.203; François Paillard et al., 'Plasma Palmitoleic Acid, a Product of Stearoyl-coA Desaturase Activity, Is an Independent Marker of Triglyceridemia and Abdominal Adiposity,' *Nutrition, Metabolism & Cardiovascular Diseases* 18, no. 6 (July 2008): 436–40, https://doi.org/10.1016/j.numecd.2007.02.017; Yuvaraj Mahendran et al., 'Association of Erythrocyte Membrane Fatty Acids with Changes in Glycemia and Risk of Type 2 Diabetes,' *The American Journal of Clinical Nutrition* 99, no. 1 (January 2014): 79–85, https://doi.org/10.3945/ajcn.113.069740; Bengt Vessby et al., 'The Risk to Develop NIDDM Is Related to the Fatty Acid Composition of the Serum Cholesterol Esters,' *Diabetes* 43, no. 11 (November 1994): 1353–7, https://doi.org/10.2337/diab.43.11.1353; Luc Djoussé et al., 'Plasma Phospholipid Concentration of Cis-Palmitoleic Acid and Risk of Heart Failure,' *Circulation: Heart Failure* 5, no. 6 (October 2012): 703–9, https://doi.org/10.1161/CIRCHEARTFAILURE.112.967802; Cassandra E. Forsythe et al., 'Comparison of Low Fat and Low Carbohydrate Diets on Circulating Fatty Acid Composition and Markers of Inflammation,' *Lipids* 43, no. 1 (January 2008), https://doi.org/10.1007/s11745-007-3132-7.

3. Yan Ni et al., 'Circulating Unsaturated Fatty Acids Delineate the Metabolic Status of Obese Individuals,' *EBioMedicine* 2, no. 10 (October 2015), https://doi.org/10.1016/j.ebiom.2015.09.004; E. Warensjö et al., 'Fatty Acid Composition of Serum Lipids Predicts the Development of the Metabolic Syndrome in Men,' *Diabetologia* 48, 1999–2005 (2005), https://doi.org/10.1007/s00125-005-1897-x; Ali H. Mokdad et al., 'The State of US Health, 1990–2016: Burden of Diseases, Injuries, and Risk Factors among US States,' *JAMA* 319, no. 14 (April 2018): 1444–72, https://doi.org/10.1001/jama.2018.0158.

4. Parker N. Hyde et al., 'Dietary Carbohydrate Restriction Improves Metabolic Syndrome Independent of Weight Loss,' *JCI Insight* 4 (June 2019), https://doi.org/10.1172/jci.insight.128308; Brittanie M. Volk et al., 'Effects of Step-Wise Increases in Dietary Carbohydrate on Circulating Saturated Fatty Acids and

Palmitoleic Acid in Adults with Metabolic Syndrome,' *PLoS One* 9, no. 11 (November 2014), https://doi.org/10.1371/journal.pone.0113605.

5. M. Murashima et al., 'Phase I Study of Multiple Biomarkers for Metabolism and Oxidative Stress after One-Week Intake of Broccoli Sprouts,' *BioFactors* 22, no. 1-4 (2004): 271–5, https://doi.org/10.1002/biof.5520220154.

6. Lingyun Wu and Bernhard H. J. Juurlink, 'The Impaired Glutathione System and Its Up-regulation by Sulforaphane in Vascular Smooth Muscle Cells from Spontaneously Hypertensive Rats,' *Journal of Hypertension* 19, no. 10 (October 2001): 1819–25, https://doi.org/10.1097/00004872-200110000-00016.

7. Raquel Villegas et al., 'Vegetable but Not Fruit Consumption Reduces the Risk of Type 2 Diabetes in Chinese Women,' *The Journal of Nutrition* 138, no. 3 (March 2008): 574–80, https://doi.org/10.1093/jn/138.3.574; Simin Liu et al., 'A Prospective Study of Fruit and Vegetable Intake and the Risk of Type 2 Diabetes in Women,' *Diabetes Care* 27, no. 12 (December 2004): 2993–6, https://doi.org/10.2337/diacare.27.12.2993.

8. K. He et al., 'Changes in Intake of Fruits and Vegetables in Relation to Risk of Obesity and Weight Gain among Middle-Aged Women,' *International Journal of Obesity* 28, no. 12 (October 2004): 1569–74, https://doi.org/10.1038/sj.ijo.0802795.

9. M. C. Morris et al., 'Associations of Vegetable and Fruit Consumption with Age-related Cognitive Change,' *Neurology* 67, no. 8 (October 2006): https://doi.org/10.1212/01.wnl.0000240224.38978.d8.

10. Tao Huang et al., 'Consumption of Whole Grains and Cereal Fiber and Total and Cause-Specific Mortality: Prospective Analysis of 367,442 Individuals,' *BMC Medicine* 13, no. 85 (April 2015), https://doi.org/10.1186/s12916-015-0338-z; Yang Yang et al., 'Association Between Dietary Fiber and Lower Risk of All-Cause Mortality: A Meta-analysis of Cohort Studies,' *American Journal of Epidemiology* 181, no. 2 (January 2015), https://doi.org/10.1093/aje/kwu257; Marc P. McRae, 'Dietary Fiber Is Beneficial for the Prevention of Cardiovascular Disease: An Umbrella Review of Meta-analyses,' *Journal of Chiropractic Medicine* 16, no. 4 (December 2017): 289–99, https://doi.org/10.1016/j.jcm.2017.05.005.

11. Lauren C. Blekkenhorst et al., 'Association of Dietary Nitrate with Atherosclerotic Vascular Disease Mortality: A Prospective Cohort Study of Older Adult Women,' *The American Journal of Clinical Nutrition* 106, no. 1 (July 2017): 207–16, https://doi.org/10.3945/ajcn.116.146761.

12. Ammar W. Ashor et al., 'Medium-Term Effects of Dietary Nitrate Supplementation on Systolic and Diastolic Blood Pressure in Adults: A Systematic Review and Meta-analysis,' *Journal of Hypertension* 35, no. 7 (July 2017): 1353–9, https://doi.org/10.1097/HJH.0000000000001305; Kristin L. Jonvik et al., 'Nitrate-Rich Vegetables Increase Plasma Nitrate and Nitrite Concentrations and Lower Blood Pressure in Healthy Adults,' *The Journal of Nutrition* 146, no. 5 (May 2016): 986–93, https://doi.org/10.3945/jn.116.229807.

13. Alex Liu et al., 'Effects of a Nitrate-Rich Meal on Arterial Stiffness and Blood Pressure in Healthy Volunteers,' *Nitric Oxide* 35 (November 2013): 123–30, https://doi.org

/10.1016/j.niox.2013.10.001; Catherine P. Bondonno et al., 'Flavonoid-Rich Apples and Nitrate-Rich Spinach Augment Nitric Oxide Status and Improve Endothelial Function in Healthy Men and Women: A Randomized Controlled Trial,' *Free Radical Biology and Medicine* 52, no. 1 (January 2012): 95–102, https://doi.org/10.1016/j.freeradbiomed.2011.09.028; Ditte A. Hobbs et al., 'Acute Ingestion of Beetroot Bread Increases Endothelium-Independent Vasodilation and Lowers Diastolic Blood Pressure in Healthy Men: A Randomized Controlled Trial,' *The Journal of Nutrition* 143, no. 9 (September 2013): 1399–1405, https://doi.org/10.3945/jn.113.175778.

14. Cindy M. T. van der Avoort et al., 'A Nitrate-Rich Vegetable Intervention Elevates Plasma Nitrate and Nitrite Concentrations and Reduces Blood Pressure in Healthy Young Adults,' *Journal of the Academy of Nutrition and Dietetics* 120, no. 8 (August 2020): 1305–17, https://doi.org/10.1016/j.jand.2020.02.014.

15. Catherine Roze Braunstein et al., 'Effect of Low-Glycemic Index/Load Diets on Body Weight: A Systematic Review and Meta-analysis,' *The FASEB Journal* 30, no. S1 (April 2016), https://doi.org/10.1096/fasebj.30.1_supplement.906.9.

16. Christine Clar et al., 'Low Glycaemic Index Diets for the Prevention of Cardiovascular Disease,' *Cochrane Database of Systematic Reviews* 7, (July 2017), https://doi.org/10.1002/14651858.cd004467.pub3.

17. Alireza Milajerdi et al., 'The Effect of Dietary Glycemic Index and Glycemic Load on Inflammatory Biomarkers: A Systematic Review and Meta-analysis of Randomized Clinical Trials,' *The American Journal of Clinical Nutrition* 107, no. 4 (April 2018): 593–606, https://doi.org/10.1093/ajcn/nqx042.

18. Mads F. Hjorth et al., 'Personalized Dietary Management of Overweight and Obesity Based on Measures of Insulin and Glucose,' *Annual Review of Nutrition* 38 (August 2018): 245–72, https://doi.org/10.1146/annurev-nutr-082117-051606.

Chapter 8: Turn The Dial on Fats

1. C. Diekman and K. Malcolm, 'Consumer Perception and Insights on Fats and Fatty Acids: Knowledge on the Quality of Diet Fat,' *Annals of Nutrition and Metabolism* 54, no. 1 (July 2009), https://doi.org/10.1159/000220824.

2. 'Australian Health Survey: Nutrition First Results – Food and Nutrients, 2011–2012,' Australian Bureau of Statistics, Canberra, September 5, 2014, https://www.abs.gov.au/statistics/health/health-conditions-and-risks/australian-health-survey-nutrition-first-results-foods-and-nutrients/latest-release; Lorraine Mitchell, 'U.S. and EU Consumption Comparisons,' Published by Economic Research Service, USDA, Washington D.C. (January 20004, WRS-04-04), https://www.ers.usda.gov/webdocs/outlooks/40408/30650_wrs0404_002.pdf?v=487.4.

3. Ramón Estruch et al., 'Primary Prevention of Cardiovascular Disease with a Mediterranean Diet,' *The New England Journal of Medicine* 368, no. 14 (April 2013): 1279–90, https://DOI:10.1056/NEJMoa1200303; Lawrence J. Appel et al., 'Effects of Protein, Monounsaturated Fat, and Carbohydrate Intake on Blood Pressure and Serum Lipids: Results of the OmniHeart Randomized Trial,' *JAMA* 294,

no. 19 (November 2005), https://doi.org/10.1001/jama.294.19.2455; Barbara V. Howard et al., 'Low-Fat Dietary Pattern and Risk of Cardiovascular Disease: The Women's Health Initiative Randomized Controlled Dietary Modification Trial,' *JAMA* 295, no. 6 (February 2006), https://doi.org/10.1001/jama.295.6.655; Leslie F. Tinker et al., 'Low-Fat Dietary Pattern and Risk of Treated Diabetes Mellitus in Postmenopausal Women: The Women's Health Initiative Randomized Controlled Dietary Modification Trial,' *Archives of Internal Medicine* 168, no. 14 (July 2008), https://doi.org/10.1001/archinte.168.14.1500; Ross L. Prentice et al., 'Low-Fat Dietary Pattern and Risk of Invasive Breast Cancer: The Women's Health Initiative Randomized Controlled Dietary Modification Trial,' *JAMA* 295, no. 6 (February 2006), https://doi.org/10.1001/jama.295.6.629; Shirley A. A. Beresford et al., 'Low-Fat Dietary Pattern and Risk of Colorectal Cancer: The Women's Health Initiative Randomized Controlled Dietary Modification Trial,' *JAMA* 295, no. 6 (February 2006), https://doi.org/10.1001/jama.295.6.643.

4. Frank B. Hu and Walter C. Willett, 'Optimal Diets for Prevention of Coronary Heart Disease,' *JAMA* 288, no. 20 (November 2002), https://doi.org/10.1001/jama.288.20.2569.

5. 'Scientific Report of the 2015 Dietary Guidelines Advisory Committee,' Dietary Guidelines Advisory Committee, Advisory Report to the Secretary of Health and Human Services and the Secretary of Agriculture 2015, accessed June 14, 2019, https://health.gov/dietaryguidelines/2015-scientific-report/.

6. Russell J. de Souza et al., 'Intake of Saturated and Trans Unsaturated Fatty Acids and Risk of all Cause Mortality, Cardiovascular Disease, and Type 2 Diabetes: Systematic Review and Meta-analysis of Observational Studies,' *BMJ* 351 (August 2015), https://doi.org/10.1136/bmj.h3978; Zoë Harcombe et al., 'Evidence from Randomised Controlled Trials Does Not Support Current Dietary Fat Guidelines: A Systematic Review and Meta-analysis,' *Open Heart* 3, no. 2 (August 2016), http://doi.org/10.1136/openhrt-2016-000409; Christopher E. Ramsden et al., 'Re-evaluation of the Traditional Diet-Heart Hypothesis: Analysis of Recovered Data from Minnesota Coronary Experiment (1968–73),' *BMJ* 353 (April 2016), https://doi.org/10.1136/bmj.i1246; Patty W. Siri-Tarino et al., 'Meta-analysis of Prospective Cohort Studies Evaluating the Association of Saturated Fat with Cardiovascular Disease,' *American Journal of Clinical Nutrition* 91, no. 3 (March 2010), https://doi.org/10.3945/ajcn.2009.27725; Lee Hooper et al., 'Reduction in Saturated Fat Intake for Cardiovascular Disease,' *Cochrane Database of Systematic Reviews* 6 (June 2015), https://doi.org/10.1002/14651858.CD011737; Dariush Mozaffarian et al., 'Effects on Coronary Heart Disease of Increasing Polyunsaturated Fat in Place of Saturated Fat: A Systematic Review and Meta-analysis of Randomized Controlled Trials,' *PLoS Medicine* 7, no.3 (March 2010), https://doi.org/10.1371/journal.pmed.1000252/.

7. Zoe Harcombe, 'US Dietary Guidelines: Is Saturated Fat a Nutrient of Concern?,' *British Journal of Sports Medicine* 53 (October 2019), https://doi.org/10.1136/bjsports-2018-099420.

8. Stephan Vanvliet et al., 'Impossible to Go Beyond Beef? A Nutriomics Comparison,' Frontiers August (2020), https:doi/10.21203/rs.3.rs-65066/v1.

9. Robert H. Eckel et al,, '2013 AHA/ACC Guideline on Lifestyle Management to Reduce Cardiovascular Risk: A Report of the American College of Cardiology/ American Heart Association Task Force on Practice Guidelines,' *Journal of the American College of Cardiology* 129, no. 25 (June 2014), https://doi.org/10.1161 /01.cir.0000437740.48606.d1.

10. Jan Borén et al., 'Low-Density Lipoproteins Cause Atherosclerotic Cardiovascular Disease: Pathophysiological, Genetic, and Therapeutic Insights: A Consensus State-ment from the European Atherosclerosis Society Consensus Panel,' *European Heart Journal* 41, no. 24 (June 2020), 2313–30, https://doi.org/10.1093/eurheartj/ehz962.

11. Brian A. Ference et al., 'Low-Density Lipoproteins Cause Atherosclerotic Cardio-vascular Disease. 1. Evidence from Genetic, Epidemiologic, and Clinical Studies. A Consensus Statement from the European Atherosclerosis Society Consensus Panel,' *European Heart Journal* 38, no. 32 (August 2017), 2459–72, https://doi.org /10.1093/eurheartj/ehx144.

12. Ronald P. Mensink et al., 'Effects of Dietary Fatty Acids and Carbohydrates on the Ratio of Serum Total to HDL Cholesterol and on Serum Lipids and Apolipo-proteins: A Meta-analysis of 60 Controlled Trials,' *The American Journal of Clinical Nutrition* 77, no. 5 (May 2003), 1146–55, https://doi.org/10.1093/ajcn/77.5.1146.

13. M. de Lorgeril et al., 'Alpha-linolenic Acid in the Prevention and Treatment of Coronary Heart Disease,' *European Heart Journal Supplements* 3, no. suppl_D (June 2001): D26–32, https://doi.org/10.1016/S1520-765X(01)90115-4; Montserrat Fitó et al., 'Effect of a Traditional Mediterranean Diet on Lipoprotein Oxidation: A Randomized Controlled Trial,' *Archives of Internal Medicine* 167, no.11 (June 2007), https://doi.org/10.1001/archinte.167.11.1195.

14. 'Spain: Coronary Heart Disease,' World Health Ranking, World Life Expectancy, accessed September 30, 2020, https://www.worldlifeexpectancy.com/spain -coronary-heart-disease#:~:text=Spain%3A%20Coronary%20Heart%20Disease &text=According%20to%20the%20latest%20WHO,Spain%20%23177%20in %20the%20world.

15. Kirsten A. Herrick et al., 'Estimating Usual Dietary Intake from National Health and Nutrition Examination Survey Data Using the National Cancer Institute Method,' (Washington, DC: National Center for Health Statistics, Vital and Health Statistics 2, no. 178, February 2018), https://www.cdc.gov/nchs/data /series/sr_02/sr02_178.pdf.

16. Lauren E. O'Connor et al., 'Total Red Meat Intake of ≥0.5 Servings/d Does Not Negatively Influence Cardiovascular Disease Risk Factors: A Systemically Searched Meta-analysis of Randomized Controlled Trials,' *The American Journal of Clinical Nutrition* 105, no. 1 (January 2017): 57–69, https://doi.org/10.3945/ajcn .116.142521; Dena Zeraatkar et al., 'Effect of Lower Versus Higher Red Meat Intake on Cardiometabolic and Cancer Outcomes: A Systematic Review of

Randomized Trials,' *Annals of Internal Medicine* 171 (November 2019), https:// doi.org/10.7326/M19-0622.

17. Lee Hooper et al., 'Effects of Chocolate, Cocoa, and Flavan-3-ols on Cardiovascular Health: A Systematic Review and Meta-analysis of Randomized Trials,' *The American Journal of Clinical Nutrition* 95, no. 3 (March 2012): 740–51, https://doi .org/10.3945/ajcn.111.023457; Lei Jia et al., 'Short-Term Effect of Cocoa Product Consumption on Lipid Profile: A Meta-analysis of Randomized Controlled Trials,' *The American Journal of Clinical Nutrition* 92, no. 1 (July 2010): 218–25, https://doi.org/10.3945/ajcn.2009.28202.

18. J. Pérez-Jiménez et al., 'Identification of the 100 Richest Dietary Sources of Polyphenols: An Application of the Phenol-Explorer Database,' *European Journal of Clinical Nutrition* 64, Supplement 3 (November 2010): S112–120, https://doi .org/10.1038/ejcn.2010.221.

19. Rinat Rivka Ran-Ressler et al., 'Branched-Chain Fatty Acid Content of Foods and Estimated Intake in the USA,' *British Journal of Nutrition* 112, no. 4 (2014): 565–72, https://doi.org/10.1017/S0007114514001081.

20. Arne Astrup, 'Yogurt and Dairy Product Consumption to Prevent Cardiometabolic Diseases: Epidemiologic and Experimental Studies,' *The American Journal of Clinical Nutrition* 99, no. 5 (April 2014): 1235S–1242, https://doi.org/10.3945 /ajcn.113.073015; Daniel B. Ibsen et al., 'Substitutions Between Dairy Product Subgroups and Risk of Type 2 Diabetes: The Danish Diet, Cancer and Health Cohort,' *British Journal of Nutrition* 118, no. 11 (November 2017): 989–97, https:// doi.org/10.1017/S0007114517002896; Andrew Mente et al., 'Association of Dietary Nutrients with Blood Lipids and Blood Pressure in 18 Countries: A Cross-sectional Analysis from the PURE Study,' *The Lancet: Diabetes & Endocrinology* 5, no. 10 (October 2017): 774–87, https://doi.org/10.1016/S2213-8587(17)30283-8.

21. Tanya Thorning et al., 'Whole Dairy Matrix or Single Nutrients in Assessment of Health Effects: Current Evidence and Knowledge Gaps,' *American Journal of Clinical Nutrition* 105 (May 2017), https://doi:10.3945/ajcn.116.151548.

22. 'Saturated Fat, Heart Disease, and Stroke,' Heart & Stroke Foundation of Canada, August 2015, accessed February 17, 2016, https://www.heartandstroke.ca/- /media/pdf-files/canada/position-statement/saturatedfat-eng-final.ashx.

23. Maria-Isabel Covas MI, et al.. 'The Effect of Polyphenols in Olive Oil on Heart Disease Risk Factors: A Randomized Trial,' *Annals of Internal Medicine* 145, no. 5 (September 2006), https://doi.org/10.7326/0003-4819-145-5-200609050-00006; Isabel Bondia-Pons et al., 'Moderate Consumption of Olive Oil by Healthy European Men Reduces Systolic Blood Pressure in Non-Mediterranean Participants,' *The Journal of Nutrition* 137, no. 1 (January 2007): 84–7, https://doi.org/10.1093/jn/137.1.84.

24. Kay-Tee Khaw et al., 'Randomised Trial of Coconut Oil, Olive Oil or Butter on Blood Lipids and Other Cardiovascular Risk Factors in Healthy Men and Women,' *BMJ Open* 8, no. 3 (March 2018), http://dx.doi.org/10.1136/bmjopen-2017-020167; Sakunthala Arunima and Thankappan Rajamohan, 'Influence of Virgin Coconut

Oil-Enriched Diet on the Transcriptional Regulation of Fatty Acid Synthesis and Oxidation in Rats – A Comparative Study,' *British Journal of Nutrition* 111, no. 10 (February 2014): 1782–90, https://doi.org/10.1017/S000711451400004X.

25. A. M. Marina et al., 'Antioxidant Capacity and Phenolic Acids of Virgin Coconut Oil,' *International Journal of Food Sciences and Nutrition* 60, Suppl 2 (2009): 114–23, https://doi.org/10.1080/09637480802549127.

26. Linia C. Del Gobbo et al., 'Are Phytosterols Responsible for the Low-Density Lipoprotein-Lowering Effects of Tree Nuts?: A Systematic Review and Meta-analysis,' *Journal of the American College of Cardiology* 65, no. 25 (June 2015): 2765–7, https://doi.org/10.1016/j.jacc.2015.03.595; Joan Sabaté et al., 'Nut Consumption and Blood Lipid Levels: A Pooled Analysis of 25 Intervention Trials,' *Archives of Internal Medicine* 170, no. 9 (May 2010): 821–7, https://doi.org/10.1001/archinternmed.2010.79.

27. Li Wang et al., 'Effect of a Moderate Fat Diet with and without Avocados on Lipoprotein Particle Number, Size and Subclasses in Overweight and Obese Adults: A Randomized, Controlled Trial,' *Journal of the American Heart Association* 4, no. 1 (January 2015), https://doi.org/10.1161/JAHA.114.001355.

28. A. P. Simopoulos, 'Evolutionary Aspects of Diet, the Omega-6/Omega-3 Ratio and Genetic Variation: Nutritional Implications for Chronic Diseases,' *Biomedicine & Pharmacotherapy* 60, no. 9 (November 2006): 502–7, https://doi.org/10.1016/j.biopha.2006.07.080.

29. Tanya L. Blasbalg et al., 'Changes in Consumption of Omega-3 and Omega-6 Fatty Acids in the United States During the 20th Century,' *The American Journal of Clinical Nutrition* 93, no. 5 (May 2011): 950–62, https://doi.org/10.3945/ajcn.110.006643.

30. 'Fats and Fatty Acids in Human Nutrition. Report of an Expert Consultation,' World Health Organization (2010), https://www.who.int/nutrition/publications/nutrientrequirements/fatsandfattyacids_humannutrition/en/.

31. Sang-Wook Yi et al., 'Association Between Fasting Glucose and All-Cause Mortality According to Sex and Age: A Prospective Cohort Study,' *Scientific Reports* 7, no. 8194 (August 2017), https://doi.org/10.1038/s41598-017-08498-6.

32. Kirk W. Beach, 'A Theoretical Model to Predict the Behavior of Glycosylated Hemoglobin Levels,' *Journal of Theoretical Biology* 81, no. 3 (December 1979), https://doi.org/10.1016/0022-5193(79)90052-3.

33. Cosimo Giannini et al., 'The Triglyceride-to-HDL Cholesterol Ratio: Association with Insulin Resistance in Obese Youths of Different Ethnic Backgrounds,' *Diabetes Care* 34, no. 8 (August 2011): 1869–74, https://doi.org/10.2337/dc10-2234; Su Jong Kim-Dorner et al., 'Should Triglycerides and the Triglycerides to High-Density Lipoprotein Cholesterol Ratio Be Used as Surrogates for Insulin Resistance?' *Metabolism* 59, no. 2(February 2010): 299–304, https://doi.org/10.1016/j.metabol.2009.07.027.

34. Mian Tian et al., 'Comparison of Apolipoprotein B/A1 Ratio, Framingham Risk Score and TC/HDL-c for Predicting Clinical Outcomes in Patients Undergoing Percutaneous Coronary Intervention,' *Lipids in Health and Disease* 18, no. 202 (November 2019), https://doi.org/10.1186/s12944-019-1144-y; Kang H. Zheng et al., 'apoB/

apoA-I Ratio and Lp(a) Associations with Aortic Valve Stenosis Incidence: Insights from the EPIC-Norfolk Prospective Population Study,' *Journal of the American Heart Association* 8, no. 16 (August 2019), https://doi.org/10.1161/JAHA.119.013020; Jiayuan Wu et al., 'Serum Apolipoprotein B-to-Apolipoprotein A1 Ratio Is Independently Associated with Disease Severity in Patients with Acute Pancreatitis,' *Scientific Reports* 9, no. 7764 (May 2019), https://doi.org/10.1038/s41598-019-44244-w.

35. Li Wang et al., 'Effect of a Moderate Fat Diet with and without Avocados on Lipoprotein Particle Number, Size and Subclasses in Overweight and Obese Adults: A Randomized, Controlled Trial,' *Journal of the American Heart Association* 4, no. 1 (January 2015), https://doi.org/10.1161/JAHA.114.001355.

Chapter 9: Leaner, Faster, Stronger

1. Joan Font-Burgada et al., 'Obesity and Cancer: The Oil that Feeds the Flame,' *Cell Metabolism* 23, no. 1 (January 2016): 48–62, https://doi.org/10.1016/j.cmet.2015.12.015; Francisco B. Ortega et al., 'Obesity and Cardiovascular Disease,' *Circulation Research* 118, no. 11 (May 2016): 1752–70, https://doi.org/10.1161/CIRCRESAHA.115.306883; Steven E. Kahn et al., 'Mechanisms Linking Obesity to Insulin Resistance and Type 2 Diabetes,' *Nature* 444, no. 7121 (December 2006): 840–6, https://doi.org/10.1038/nature05482.

2. James R. Cerhan et al., 'A Pooled Analysis of Waist Circumference and Mortality in 650,000 Adults,' *Mayo Clinic Proceedings* 89, no. 3 (March 2014): 335–45, https://doi.org/10.1016/j.mayocp.2013.11.011; Lawrence de Koning et al., 'Waist Circumference and Waist-to-Hip Ratio as Predictors of Cardiovascular Events: Meta-regression Analysis of Prospective," *European Heart Journal* 28, no. 7 (April 2007): 850–6, https://doi.org/10.1093/eurheartj/ehm026; A. E. Staiano et al., 'Body Mass Index Versus Waist Circumference as Predictors of Mortality in Canadian Adults,' *International Journal of Obesity* 36, no. 11 (January 2012): 1450–4, https://doi.org/10.1038/ijo.2011.268.

3. Barbara Riegel et al., 'Self-Care for the Prevention and Management of Cardiovascular Disease and Stroke: A Scientific Statement for Healthcare Professionals from the American Heart Association,' *Journal of the American Heart Association* 6, no. 9 (August 2017), https://doi.org/10.1161/JAHA.117.006997; Antero Kesäniemi et al., 'Advancing the Future of Physical Activity Guidelines in Canada: An Independent Expert Panel Interpretation of the Evidence,' *International Journal of Behavioral Nutrition and Physical Activity* 7, no. 41 (May 2010), https://doi.org/10.1186/1479-5868-7-41; 'Global Status Report on Noncommunicable Diseases 2014,' World Health Organization (2014), https://www.who.int/nmh/publications/ncd-status-report-2014/en/; Clinton A. Brawner et al., 'Prevalence of Physical Activity Is Lower Among Individuals with Chronic Disease,' *Medicine & Science in Sports & Exercise* 48, no.6 (June 2016): 1062–7, https://doi.org/10.1249/MSS.0000000000000861.

4. Sherry L. Murphy et al., 'Deaths: Final Data for 2015,' *National Vital Statistics Report* 66, no. 6 (November 2017), https://www.cdc.gov/nchs/data/nvsr/nvsr66/nvsr66

_06.pdf; Scott A. Lear et al., 'The Effect of Physical Activity on Mortality and Cardiovascular Disease in 130,000 People from 17 High-Income, Middle-Income, and Low-Income Countries: The PURE Study,' *The Lancet* 390, no. 10113 (December 2017): 2643–54, https://doi.org/10.1016/S0140-6736(17)31634-3.

5. B. K. Pedersen and B. Saltin, 'Exercise as Medicine – Evidence for Prescribing Exercise as Therapy in 26 Different Chronic Diseases,' *Scandinavian Journal of Medicine & Science in Sports* 25, no. S3 (November 2015), https://doi.org/10.1111/sms.12581.

6. Scott A. Lear et al., 'The Effect of Physical Activity on Mortality and Cardiovascular Disease in 130,000 People from 17 High-Income, Middle-Income, and Low-Income Countries: The PURE Study,' *The Lancet* 390, no. 10113 (December 2017): 2643–54, https://doi.org/10.1016/S0140-6736(17)31634-3; Pedersen, 'Exercise as Medicine.'

7. 'Physical Activity: Adult,' World Health Organization, accessed August 3, 2019, https://www.who.int/news-room/fact-sheets/detail/physical-activity.

8. Heleen Spittaels et al., 'Objectively Measured Sedentary Time and Physical Activity Time Across the Lifespan: A Cross-Sectional Study in Four Age Groups,' *International Journal of Behavioral Nutrition and Physical Activity* 9, no. 149 (December 2012), https://doi.org/10.1186/1479-5868-9-149.

9. Anatoli Petridou et al., 'Exercise in the Management of Obesity,' *Metabolism* 92 (March 2019): 163–9, https://doi.org/10.1016/j.metabol.2018.10.009; Lance E. Davidson et al., 'Effects of Exercise Modality on Insulin Resistance and Functional Limitation in Older Adults: A Randomized Controlled Trial,' *Archives of Internal Medicine* 169, no. 2 (January 2009): 122–31, https://doi.org/10.1001/archinternmed.2008.558; Dorth Stensvold et al., 'Strength Training Versus Aerobic Interval Training to Modify Risk Factors of Metabolic Syndrome,' *Journal of Applied Physiology* 108, no. 4 (April 2010), https://doi.org/10.1152/japplphysiol.00996.2009; Suleen S. Ho et al., 'Resistance, Aerobic, and Combination Training on Vascular Function in Overweight and Obese Adults,' *The Journal of Clinical Hypertension* 14, no. 12 (August 2012), https://doi.org/10.1111/j.1751-7176.2012.00700.x; Suleen S. Ho et al., 'The Effect of 12 Weeks of Aerobic, Resistance or Combination Exercise Training on Cardiovascular Risk Factors in the Overweight and Obese in a Randomized Trial,' *BMC Public Health* 12, no. 704 (August 2012), https://doi.org/10.1186/1471-2458-12-704; I. Ismail et al., 'A Systematic Review and Meta-analysis of the Effect of Aerobic vs. Resistance Training on Visceral Fat,' *Obesity Reviews* 13, no. 1 (September 2011), https://doi.org/10.1111/j.1467-789X.2011.00931.x; Elizabeth C. Schroeder et al., 'Comparative Effectiveness of Aerobic, Resistance and Combined Training on Cardiovascular Disease Risk Factors: A Randomized Controlled Trial,' *PLoS ONE* 14, no. 1 (January 2019), https://doi.org/10.1371/journal.pone.0210292; James E. Clark, 'Diet, Exercise or Diet with Exercise: Comparing the Effectiveness of Treatment Options for Weight-Loss and Changes in Fitness for Adults (18-65 Years Old) Who Are Overfat, or Obese; Systematic Review and Meta-analysis,' *Journal of Diabetes & Metabolic Disorders* 14, no. 31 (April 2015), https://doi.org/10.1186

/s40200-015-0154-1; Adrian Thorogood et al., 'Isolated Aerobic Exercise and Weight Loss: A Systematic Review and Meta-analysis of Randomized Controlled Trials,' *The American Journal of Medicine* 124, no. 8 (August 2011): 747–55, https://doi.org/10.1016/j.amjmed.2011.02.037.

10. Petros C. Dinas et al., 'Exercise-Induced Biological and Psychological Changes in Overweight and Obese Individuals: A Review of Recent Evidence,' *International Scholarly Research Notices* (February 2014), https://doi.org/10.1155/2014 /964627; Eliane Aparecida Castro et al., 'What Is the Most Effective Exercise Protocol to Improve Cardiovascular Fitness in Overweight and Obese Subjects?' *Journal of Sport and Health Science* 6, no. 4 (December 2017): 454–61, https://doi .org/10.1016/j.jshs.2016.04.007.

11. Kornanong Yuenyongchaiwat et al., 'Increasing Walking Steps Daily Can Reduce Blood Pressure and Diabetes in Overweight Participants,' *Diabetology International* 9, no. 1 (February 2018): 75–9, https://doi.org/10.1007/s13340-017-0333-z.

12. Mathias Reid-Larsen et al., 'Bicycling and All-Cause Mortality among Individuals with Diabetes,' EASD Virtual Meeting, Oral Presentation 194, Session: OP 33 (September 2020), https://www.easd.org/virtualmeeting/home.html#!resources /bicycling-and-all-cause-mortality-among-individuals-with-diabetes.

13. Jenna B. Gillen et al., 'Twelve Weeks of Sprint Interval Training Improves Indices of Cardiometabolic Health Similar to Traditional Endurance Training despite a Five-Fold Lower Exercise Volume and Time Commitment,' *PLoS One* 11, no. 4 (April 2016), https://doi.org/10.1371/journal.pone.0154075.

14. Y Lai, 'Association between Exercise Capacity and All-Cause Mortality in People with Type-2 Diabetes,' *EASD 56th Annual Meeting* (2020), Session A, 267.

15. Felipe Mattioni Maturana et al., 'Effectiveness of HIIE versus MICT in Improving Cardiometabolic Risk Factors in Health and Disease: A Meta-analysis,' *Medicine & Science in Sports & Exercise* (September 2020), https://doi.org/10.1249/MSS .0000000000002506.

16. Robin Poole et al., 'Coffee Consumption and Health: Umbrella Review of Meta-analyses of Multiple Health Outcomes,' *BMJ* 359 (November 2017), https://doi .org/10.1136/bmj.j5024.

17. Ronald J. Maughan et al., 'IOC Consensus Statement: Dietary Supplements and the High-Performance Athlete,' *British Journal of Sports Medicine* 52, no. 7 (2018): 439–55, https://doi.org/10.1136/bjsports-2018-099027.

18. Giuseppe Grosso et al., 'Coffee Consumption and Risk of All-Cause, Cardiovascular, and Cancer Mortality in Smokers and Non-smokers: A Dose-Response Meta-analysis,' *European Journal of Epidemiology* 31, no. 12 (October 2016): 1191–205, https://doi.org/10.1007/s10654-016-0202-2.

19. Habib Yarizadeh et al., 'The Effect of Aerobic and Resistance Training and Combined Exercise Modalities on Subcutaneous Abdominal Fat: A Systematic Review and Meta-analysis of Randomized Clinical Trials,' *Advances in Nutrition* (August 2020), https://doi.org/10.1093/advances/nmaa090.

20. James R. Cerhan et al., 'A Pooled Analysis of Waist Circumference and Mortality in 650,000 Adults,' *Mayo Clinic Proceedings* 89, no. 3 (March 2014): 335–45, https://doi.org/10.1016/j.mayocp.2013.11.011; Lawrence de Koning et al., 'Waist Circumference and Waist-to-Hip Ratio as Predictors of Cardiovascular Events: Meta-regression Analysis of Prospective,' *European Heart Journal* 28, no. 7 (April 2007): 850–6, https://doi.org/10.1093/eurheartj/ehm026; A. E. Staiano et al., 'Body Mass Index versus Waist Circumference as Predictors of Mortality in Canadian Adults,' *International Journal of Obesity (Lond)* 36, no. 11 (November 2012):1450–4, https://doi.org/10.1038/ijo.2011.268.

21. Brad J. Schoenfeld, *Science and Development of Muscle Hypertrophy* (Champaign, IL: Human Kinetics, 2016), 29–41.

22. Brad Schoenfeld, 'Maximize Hypertrophy Training, Fat Loss Myths and Nutrition for Building Muscle,' interview with Dr Marc Bubbs, *Dr. Bubbs Performance Podcast*, June 22, 2017, https://www.athleteevolution.org/podcast-episodes/2017/6/building-muscle-burning-fat-and-evidenced-based-nutrition-w-dr-brad-schoenfeld.

23. Brad J. Schoenfeld et al., 'Strength and Hypertrophy Adaptations Between Low- vs. High-Load Resistance Training: A Systematic Review and Meta-analysis,' *Journal of Strength and Conditioning Research* 31, no. 12 (December 2017): 3508–23, https://doi.org/10.1519/jsc.0000000000002200.

24. Barbara Strasser and Wolfgang Schobersberger, 'Evidence for Resistance Training as a Treatment Therapy in Obesity,' *Journal of Obesity* 2011, no. 7 (August 2010): 1-9, https://dx.doi.org/10.1155/2011/482564.

25. Brad J. Schoenfeld et al., 'Dose-Response Relationship between Weekly Resistance Training Volume and Increases in Muscle Mass: A Systematic Review and Meta-analysis,' *Journal of Sports Sciences* 35, no. 11 (2017), https://doi.org/10.1080/02640414.2016.1210197.

26. Brett R. Gordon et al., 'Association of Efficacy of Resistance Exercise Training with Depressive Symptoms: Meta-analysis and Meta-regression Analysis of Randomized Clinical Trials,' *JAMA Psychiatry* 75, no. 6 (June 2018): 566–76, https://doi.org/10.1001/jamapsychiatry.2018.0572.

27. Matheus Pelinski da Silveira et al., 'Physical Exercise as a Tool to Help the Immune System Against COVID-19: An Integrative Review of the Current Literature,' *Clinical and Experimental Medicine* 6 (July 2020), https://doi.org/10.1007/s10238-020-00650-3.

Chapter 10: Recovery Starts with Sleep

1. Michael A. Grandner et al., 'Mortality Associated with Short Sleep Duration: The Evidence, the Possible Mechanisms, and the Future,' *Sleep Medicine Reviews* 14, no. 3 (June 2010): 191–203, https://doi.org/10.1016/j.smrv.2009.07.006.

2. S. Fenton et al., 'The Influence of Sleep Health on Dietary Intake: A Systematic Review and Meta-analysis of Intervention Studies,' *Journal of Human Nutrition & Dietetics* (October 2020), https://doi.org/10.1111/jhn.12813.

3. S. Hakki Onen et al., 'The Effects of Total Sleep Deprivation, Selective Sleep Interruption and Sleep Recovery on Pain Tolerance Thresholds in Healthy Subjects,' *Journal of Sleep Research* 10, no. 1 (July 2008), https://doi.org/10.1046/j.1365 -2869.2001.00240.x.

4. Matthew D. Milewski et al., 'Chronic Lack of Sleep Is Associated with Increased Sports Injuries in Adolescent Athletes,' *Journal of Pediatric Orthopaedics* 34, no. 2 (March 2014): 129–33, https://doi.org/10.1097/BPO.0000000000000151.

5. Hugh H. K. Fullagar et al., 'Sleep and Athletic Performance: The Effects of Sleep Loss on Exercise Performance, and Physiological and Cognitive Responses to Exercise,' *Sports Medicine* 45, no. 2 (2015), https://doi.org/10.1007/s40279-014-0260-0.

6. Shalini Paruthi et al., 'Consensus Statement of the American Academy of Sleep Medicine on the Recommended Amount of Sleep for Healthy Children: Methodology and Discussion,' *Journal of Clinical Sleep Medicine* 12, no. 11 (2016), http:// dx.doi.org/10.5664/jcsm.6288.

7. Michael A. Grandner et al., 'Mortality Associated with Short Sleep Duration: The Evidence, the Possible Mechanisms, and the Future,' *Sleep Medicine Reviews* 14, no. 3 (June 2010): 191–203, https://doi.org/10.1016/j.smrv.2009.07.006.

8. Sheldon Cohen et al., 'Sleep Habits and Susceptibility to the Common Cold,' *Archives of Internal Medicine* 169, no. 1 (January 2009), https://doi.org/10.1001 /archinternmed.2008.505.

9. Harry A. Smith et al., 'Glucose Control upon Waking Is Unaffected by Hourly Sleep Fragmentation during the Night, but Is Impaired by Morning Caffeinated Coffee,' *British Journal of Nutrition* 124, no. 10 (June 2020), https://doi.org/10 .1017/S0007114520001865.

10. Pierrick J. Arnal et al., 'Sleep Extension before Sleep Loss: Effects on Performance and Neuromuscular Function,' *Medicine & Science in Sports & Exercise* 48, no. 8 (August 2016): 1595–603, https://doi.org/10.1249/MSS.0000000000000925.

11. Norah Simpson, 'Impacts of Sleep Loss on Pain, Injury-Risk, & Neurocognition,' Interview with Dr Marc Bubbs, *The Performance Nutrition Podcast*, October 26, 2018, https://soundcloud.com/drbubbs/s2e41-impacts-of-sleep-loss-on-pain -injury-risk-neurocognition-norah-simpson.

12. Hans P. A. Van Dongen et al., 'Systematic Interindividual Differences in Neurobehavioral Impairment from Sleep Loss: Evidence of Trait-Like Differential Vulnerability,' *Sleep* 27, no. 3 (May 2004): 423–33, https://pubmed.ncbi.nlm.nih.gov/15164894/.

13. Neil P. Walsh et al., 'Position Statement. Part One: Immune Function and Exercise,' *Exercise Immunology Review* 17 (2011): 6–63.

14. Cheng-Shiun He et al., 'Is There an Optimal Vitamin D Status for Immunity in Athletes and Military Personnel?' *Exercise Immunology Review* 22 (January 2016): 41–62; Tanya M. Halliday et al., 'Vitamin D Status Relative to Diet, Lifestyle, Injury, and Illness in College Athletes,' *Medicine & Science in Sports & Exercise* 43, no. 2 (February 2011): 335–43, https://doi.org/10.1249/mss.0b013e3181eb9d4d; Cheng-Shiun He et al., 'Influence of Vitamin D Status on Respiratory Infection

Incidence and Immune Function during 4 Months of Winter Training in Endurance Sport Athletes,' *Exercise Immunology Review* 19 (2013): 86–101.

15. Hugh H. K. Fullagar et al., 'Sleep and Athletic Performance: The Effects of Sleep Loss on Exercise Performance, and Physiological and Cognitive Responses to Exercise,' *Sports Medicine* 45, no. 2 (2015): 161–86, https://doi.org/10.1007/s40279-014-0260-0.

16. Charles F. P. George et al., 'Sleep and Breathing in Professional Football Players,' *Sleep Medicine* 4, no. 4 (July 2003): 317–25, https://doi.org/10.1016/S1389 -9457(03)00113-8.

17. S. B. R. Fagundes et al., 'Prevalence of Restless Legs Syndrome in Runners,' *Sleep Medicine* 13, no. 6 (June 2012): 771, https://doi.org/10.1016/j.sleep.2012.01.001.

18. Tracey L. Sletten et al., 'Efficacy of Melatonin with Behavioural Sleep-Wake Scheduling for Delayed Sleep-Wake Phase Disorder: A Double-Blind, Randomised Clinical Trial,' *PLoS Medicine* 185, no. 6 (June 2018), https://doi.org/10.1371/journal.pmed.1002587.

19. Eric Matheson and Barry L. Hainer, 'Insomnia: Pharmacologic Therapy,' *American Family Physician* 96, no. 1 (July 2017): 29–35, https://www.aafp.org/afp/2017 /0701/p29.html.

20. Harri Hemilä, 'Vitamin C and Infections,' *Nutrients* 9, no. 4 (March 2017), https://doi.org/10.3390/nu9040339.

21. Harri Hemilä and Elizabeth Chalker, 'Vitamin C for Preventing and Treating the Common Cold,' *Cochrane Database of Systematic Reviews* 1 (January 2013), https://doi.org/10.1002/14651858.CD000980.pub4.

22. Stéphane François Bermon et al., 'Consensus Statement: Immunonutrition and Exercise,' *Exercise Immunology Review* 23 (February 2017).

23. Qiukui Hao, Bi Rong Dong, and Taixiang Wu, 'Probiotics for Preventing Acute Upper Respiratory Tract Infections,' *Cochrane Database of Systematic Reviews*, no. 2 (February 2015), https://doi.org/10.1002/14651858.cd006895.pub3.

24. Nicholas P. West et al., 'Probiotic Supplementation for Respiratory and Gastrointestinal Illness Symptoms in Healthy Physically Active Individuals,' *Clinical Nutrition* 33, no. 4 (August 2014): 581–7, https://doi.org/10.1016/j.clnu.2013.10.002.

25. Harri Hemilä, 'Zinc Lozenges May Shorten the Duration of Colds: A Systematic Review,' *The Open Respiratory Medicine Journal* 5, no. 1 (2011): 51–8, https://doi .org/10.2174/1874306401105010051.

Chapter 11: Recovery Strategies

1. Steven E. Kahn et al., 'Mechanisms Linking Obesity to Insulin Resistance and Type 2 Diabetes," *Nature* 444, no. 7121 (December 2006): 840–6, https://doi.org /10.1038/nature05482.

2. R. T. Claridge, *Hydropathy, or The Cold Water Cure, as Practised by Vincent Priessnitz, at Graefenberg, Silesia, Austria,* 8th ed., (London: James Madden and Co., 1843).

3. J. DeRose Evans, *A Companion to the Archaeology of the Roman Republic,* (Hoboken: Wiley-Blackwell, 2013).

4. Clare M. Eglin et al., 'Previous Recreational Cold Exposure Does Not Alter Endothelial Function or Sensory Thermal Thresholds in the Hands or Feet,' *Experimental Physiology* 106, no. 1 (May 2020), https://doi.org/10.1113/EP088555.

5. Mike Tipton, 'Extreme Environmental Physiology: Life at the Limits,' *Physiology News* (April 2019): 19, https://doi.org/10.36866/pn.114.19.

6. Hitoshi Wakabayashi et al., 'The Effect of Repeated Mild Cold Water Immersions on the Adaptation of the Vasomotor Responses,' *International Journal of Biometeorology* 56, no. 4 (2012): 631–7, https://doi.org/10.1007/s00484-011-0462-1; Sebastion Kilch et al., 'Effect of Short-Term Cold-Water Immersion on Muscle Pain Sensitivity in Elite Track Cyclists,' *Physical Therapy in Sport* 32 (July 2018), https://doi:10.1016/j.ptsp.2018.04.022.

7. Tom Mole and Pieter Mackeith, 'Cold Forced Open-Water Swimming: A Natural Intervention to Improve Postoperative Pain and Mobilisation Outcomes?" BMJ Case Reports (February 2018), http://dx.doi.org/10.1136/bcr-2017-222236.

8. Jonathan Leeder et al., 'Cold Water Immersion and Recovery from Strenuous Exercise: A Meta-analysis,' *British Journal of Sports Medicine* 46, no. 4 (2012), https://doi.org/10.1136/bjsports-2011-090061.

9. Wigand Poppendieck et al., 'Does Cold-Water Immersion after Strength Training Attenuate Training Adaptation?' *International Journal of Sports Physiology and Performance* 20 (2020), https://doi.org/10.1123/ijspp.2019-0965.

10. Mike Tipton, 'Extreme Environmental Physiology: Life at the Limits,' The Physiological Society (April 2019), https://DOI.org/10.36866/pn.114.19.

11. Karin Kraft, 'Complementary/Alternative Medicine in the Context of Prevention of Disease and Maintenance of Health,' *Preventive Medicine* 49, no. 2–3 (August–September 2009): 88–92, https://doi.org/10.1016/j.ypmed.2009.05.003.

12. Christophe Hausswirth et al., 'Effects of Whole-Body Cryotherapy vs. Far-Infrared vs. Passive Modalities on Recovery from Exercise-Induced Muscle Damage in Highly-Trained Runners,' *PLoS ONE* 6, no. 12 (December 2011), https://doi.org/10.1371/journal.pone.0027749; B. Fonda and N. Sarabon, 'Effects of Whole-Body Cryotherapy on Recovery after Hamstring Damaging Exercise: A Crossover Study,' *Scandinavian Journal of Medicine & Science in Sports* 23, no. 5 (April 2013), https://doi.org/10.1111/sms.12074.

13. J. T. Costello et al., 'Effects of Whole Body Cryotherapy and Cold Water Immersion on Knee Skin Temperature,' *International Journal of Sports Medicine* 35, no. 1 (2014): 35–40, https://doi.org/10.1055/s-0033-1343410.

14. Laura J. Wilson et al., 'Recovery Following a Marathon: A Comparison of Cold Water Immersion, Whole Body Cryotherapy and a Placebo Control,' *European Journal of Applied Physiology* 118, no. 1 (2018): 153–63, https://doi.org/10.1007/s00421-017-3757-z.

15. Nathan G. Versey et al., 'Water Immersion Recovery for Athletes: Effect on Exercise Performance and Practical Recommendations,' *Sports Medicine* 43, no. 11 (June 2013): 1101–30, https://doi.org/10.1007/s40279-013-0063-8.

16. Arianne P. Verhagen et al., 'Balneotherapy (or Spa Therapy) for Rheumatoid Arthritis,' *Cochrane Database of Systematic Reviews* 4 (2015), https://doi.org/10.1002/14651858 .CD000518.pub2; Julia Bidonde et al., 'Aquatic Exercise Training for Fibromyalgia,' *Cochrane Database of Systematic Reviews* 10 (2014), https://doi.org/10.1002/14651858 .CD011336; Jan Mehrholz et al., 'Water-Based Exercises for Improving Activities of Daily Living after Stroke,' *Cochrane Database of Systematic Reviews* 1 (2011), https:// doi.org/10.1002/14651858.CD008186.pub2; Elsa Marie Bartels et al,. 'Aquatic Exercise for the Treatment of Knee and Hip Osteoarthritis,' *Cochrane Database of Systematic Reviews* 3 (2016), https://doi.org/10.1002/14651858.CD005523.pub3.

17. Vienna E. Brunt et al., 'Passive Heat Therapy Improves Endothelial Function, Arterial Stiffness and Blood Pressure in Sedentary Humans,' *The Journal of Physiology* 594, no. 18 (June 2016), https://doi.org/10.1113/JP272453; S. P. Hoekstra et al., 'Acute and Chronic Effects of Hot Water Immersion on Inflammation and Metabolism in Sedentary, Overweight Adults,' *Journal of Applied Physiology* 125, no. 6 (December 2018), https://doi.org/10.1152/japplphysiol.00407.2018; Tanjaniina Laukkanen et al., 'Association Between Sauna Bathing and Fatal Cardiovascular and All-Cause Mortality Events,' *JAMA Intern Med.* 175, no. 4 (April 2015): 542–8, https://doi.org/10.1001/jamainternmed.2014.8187.

18. Masakuza Imamura et al., 'Repeated Thermal Therapy Improves Impaired Vascular Endothelial Function in Patients with Coronary Risk Factors,' *Journal of American College of Cardiology* 38, no. 4 (October 2001): 1083–8, https://doi.org /10.1016/S0735-1097(01)01467-X.

19. Jason Chung et al., 'HSP72 Protects Against Obesity-Induced Insulin Resistance,' *PNAS* 5, no. 105 (2008), https://doi.org/10.1073/pnas.0705799105; Philip L. Hooper, 'Hot-Tub Therapy for Type 2 Diabetes Mellitus,' *The New England Journal of Medicine* 341 (September 1999): 924–5, https://doi.org/10.1056/NEJM 199909163411216; S. P. Hoekstra et al., 'Acute and Chronic Effects of Hot Water Immersion on Inflammation and Metabolism in Sedentary, Overweight Adults,' *Journal of Applied Physiology* 125, no. 6 (December 2018): 2008–18, https://doi .org/10.1152/japplphysiol.00407.2018.

20. Keiichi Koshinaka et al., 'Elevation of Muscle Temperature Stimulates Muscle Glucose Uptake in Vivo and in Vitro' *Journal of Physiological Sciences* 63 (July 2013): 409–18, https://doi.org/10.1007/s12576-013-0278-3.

21. Scott T. Chiesa et al., 'Temperature and Blood Flow Distribution in the Human Leg during Passive Heat Stress,' *Journal of Applied Physiology* 120, no. 9 (May 2016): 1047–58, https://doi.org/10.1152/japplphysiol.00965.2015.

22. Joanna Vaile et al., 'Effect of Hydrotherapy on Signs and Symptoms of Delayed Onset Muscle Soreness,' *European Journal of Applied Physiology* 103, no. 1 (January 2008): 121–2, https://doi.org/10.1007/s00421-007-0653-y.

23. Akinori Masuda A et al., 'Repeated Thermal Therapy Diminishes Appetite Loss and Subjective Complaints in Mildly Depressed Patients,' *Psychosomatic Medicine* 4, no. 67 (2005), https://doi:10.1097/01.psy.0000171812.67767.8f.

24. Nathan G. Versey et al., 'Water Immersion Recovery for Athletes: Effect on Exercise Performance and Practical Recommendations,' *Sports Medicine* 43, no. 11 (June 2013): 1101–30, https://doi.org/10.1007/s40279-013-0063-8.

25. C. Byrne et al., 'Characteristics of Isometric and Dynamic Strength Loss following Eccentric Exercise-Induced Muscle Damage,' *Scandinavian Journal of Medicine & Science in Sports* 11, no. 3 (2001), https://doi.org/10.1046/j.1524-4725.2001.110302.x; S. M. Marcora and A. Bosio, 'Effect of Exercise-Induced Muscle Damage on Endurance Running Performance in Humans,' *Scandinavian Journal of Medicine & Science in Sports* 17, no. 6 (March 2007), https://doi.org/10.1111/j.1600-0838.2006.00627.x; Craig Twist and Roger G. Eston, 'The Effect of Exercise-Induced Muscle Damage on Perceived Exertion and Cycling Endurance Performance,' *European Journal of Applied Physiology* 105, no. 4 (2009): 559–67, https://doi.org/10.1007/s00421-008 -0935-z; Vassilis Paschalis et al., 'Eccentric Exercise Affects the Upper Limbs More than the Lower Limbs in Position Sense and Reaction Angle,' *Journal of Sports Sciences* 28, no. 1 (2010): 33–43, https://doi.org/10.1080/02640410903334764.

26. Jonathan D. Buckley et al., 'Supplementation with a Whey Protein Hydrolysate Enhances Recovery of Muscle Force-Generating Capacity following Eccentric Exercise,' *Journal of Science and Medicine in Sport* 13, no. 1 (January 2010): 178–81, https://doi.org/10.1016/j.jsams.2008.06.007; Kazunori Nosaka et al., 'Effects of Amino Acid Supplementation on Muscle Soreness and Damage,' *International Journal of Sport Nutrition and Exercise Metabolism* 16, no. 6 (2006): 620–35, https:// doi.org/10.1123/ijsnem.16.6.620.

27. Robert D. Hyldahl et al., 'Satellite Cell Activity Is Differentially Affected by Contraction Mode in Human Muscle following a Work-Matched Bout of Exercise,' *Frontiers in Physiology* 5, no. 485 (December 2014), https://doi.org/10.3389/fphys .2014.00485.

28. Tyler Barker et al., 'Vitamin D Sufficiency Associates with an Increase in Anti-inflammatory Cytokines after Intense Exercise in Humans,' *Cytokine* 65, no. 2 (February 2014): 134–7, https://doi.org/10.1016/j.cyto.2013.12.004; Kentz S. Willis et al., 'Vitamin D Status and Biomarkers of Inflammation in Runners,' *Journal of Sports Medicine* 3 (March 2012): 35–42, https://doi.org/10.2147/OAJSM.S31022.

29. Steen Olsen et al., 'Creatine Supplementation Augments the Increase in Satellite Cell and Myonuclei Number in Human Skeletal Muscle Induced by Strength Training,' *Journal of Physiology* 573, no. 2 (May 2006), https://doi.org/10.1113 /jphysiol.2006.107359.

30. Frank M. DiLorenzo et al., 'Docosahexaenoic Acid Effects Markers of Inflammation and Muscle Damage after Eccentric Exercise,' *Journal of Strength and Conditioning Research* 28, no. 10 (October 2014): 2768–74, https://doi.org/10.1519 /JSC.0000000000000617; Patrick Gray et al., 'Fish Oil Supplementation Reduces Markers of Oxidative Stress but Not Muscle Soreness after Eccentric Exercise,' *International Journal of Sport Nutrition and Exercise Metabolism* 24, no. 2 (2014): 206–14, https://doi.org/10.1123/ijsnem.2013-0081; Kelly B. Jouris et al., 'The

Effect of Omega-3 Fatty Acid Supplementation on the Inflammatory Response to Eccentric Strength Exercise,' *Journal of Sports Science & Medicine* 10, no. 3 (September 2011): 432–38, https://pubmed.ncbi.nlm.nih.gov/24150614/.

31. Rob Hodgetts, 'The Open 2013: Phil Mickelson Cards Superb 66 to Win at Muirfield,' BBC Sport, updated July 21, 2013, https://www.bbc.com/sport /golf/23397191.

32. 'Phil Mickelson on How a Bad Diet Led to Him Developing Arthritis and How his New Regime Is Paying Off,' Paul Ryding, *South China Morning Post*, accessed on December 3, 2020, https://www.scmp.com/sport/golf/article/3034019/phil -mickelson-how-bad-diet-led-him-developing-arthritis-and-how-his-new.

Chapter 12: Traits, Values and Skills

1. Bryce Tully, 'Mindset: Where Values, Skills & Traits Connect,' *The Performance Nutrition Podcast,* Interview with Dr Marc Bubbs, April 21, 2020, https://www .athleteevolution.org/podcast-season-4/s4e8-mindset-where-values-skills-amp -traits-connect-w-bryce-tully-ms.

2. Irving M. Becker and Joseph G. Rosenfeld, 'Rational Emotive Therapy – A Study of Initial Therapy Sessions of Albert Ellis,' *Psychotherapeutic Processes* 32, no. 4 (October 1976), https://doi.org/10.1002/1097-4679(197610)32:4<872::AID -JCLP2270320431>3.0.CO;2-9.

3. William F. Hart, *Life, Leadership and the Pursuit of Happiness,* (Victoria, Canada: Trafford Publishing, 2010).

4. James N. Donald and Paul W. B. Atkins, 'Mindfulness and Coping with Stress: Do Levels of Perceived Stress Matter?' *Mindfulness* 7, no. 6 (July 2016): 1423–36, https:// doi.org/10.1007/s12671-016-0584-y; Carina Remmers et al., 'Why Being Mindful May Have More Benefits Than You Realize: Mindfulness Improves Both Explicit and Implicit Mood Regulation,' *Mindfulness* 7, no. 4 (April 2016): 829–37, https:// doi.org/10.1007/s12671-016-0520-1; Ana Costa and Thorsten Barnhofer, 'Turning Towards or Turning Away: A Comparison of Mindfulness Meditation and Guided Imagery Relaxation in Patients with Acute Depression,' *Behavioural and Cognitive Psychotherapy* 44, no. 4 (2016): 410–19, https://doi.org/10.1017/S1352465815000387.

5. Lianne M. Tomfohr et al., 'Trait Mindfulness Is Associated with Blood Pressure and Interleukin-6: Exploring Interactions among Subscales of the Five Facet Mindfulness Questionnaire to Better Understand Relationships between Mindfulness and Health,' *Journal of Behavioral Medicine* 38, no. 1 (2015): 28–38, https://doi.org /10.1007/s10865-014-9575-4; Eric B. Loucks et al., 'Positive Associations of Dispositional Mindfulness with Cardiovascular Health: The New England Family Study,' *International Journal of Behavioral Medicine* 22, no. 4 (2015): 540–50, https://doi.org/10.1007/s12529-014-9448-9; Jeffrey M. Rogers et al., 'Mindfulness-Based Interventions for Adults Who Are Overweight or Obese: A Meta-analysis of Physical and Psychological Health Outcomes,' *Obesity Review* 18, no. 1 (January 2017): 51–67, https://doi.org/10.1111/obr.12461.

6. Sanjay Srivastava et al., 'Optimism in Close Relationships: How Seeing Things in a Positive Light Makes Them So,' *Journal of Personality and Social Psychology* 91, no. 1 (2006): 143–53, https://doi.org/10.1037/0022-3514.91.1.143.

7. Lauren B. Alloy et al., 'Prospective Incidence of First Onsets and Recurrences of Depression in Individuals at High and Low Cognitive Risk for Depression,' *Journal of Abnormal Psychology* 115, no. 1 (2006): 145–56, https://doi.org/10.1037/0021 -843X.115.1.145; Aimee Ellicott et al., 'Life Events and the Course of Bipolar Disorder,' *The American Journal of Psychiatry* 147, no. 9 (1990): 1194-8, https:// doi.org/10.1176/ajp.147.9.1194; Charles S. Carver and Michael F. Scheier, 'Dispositional Optimism,' *Trends in Cognitive Sciences* 18, no. 6 (June 2014): 293–9, https://doi.org/10.1016/j.tics.2014.02.003.

8. Robert Finlay-Jones and George W. Brown, 'Types of Stressful Life Event and the Onset of Anxiety and Depressive Disorders,' *Psychological Medicine* 11, no. 4 (1981): 803–15, https://doi.org/10.1017/S0033291700041301.

9. Edward C. Chang et al., 'An Examination of Optimism/Pessimism and Suicide Risk in Primary Care Patients: Does Belief in a Changeable Future Make a Difference?,' *Cognitive Therapy and Research* 37 (2013): 796–804, https://doi.org /10.1007/s10608-012-9505-0; J. S. House et al., 'Social Relationships and Health,' *Science* 241, no. 4865 (1988): 540–5, https://doi.org/10.1126/science.3399889; Vincent Lorant et al., 'Socioeconomic Inequalities in Depression: A Meta-analysis,' *American Journal of Epidemiology* 157, no. 2 (January 2003): 98-112, https://doi.org/10.1093/aje/kwf182; Ichiro Kawachi and Lisa F. Berkman, 'Social Ties and Mental Health,' *Journal of Urban Health* 78 (2001): 458–67, https://doi .org/10.1093/jurban/78.3.458.

Chapter 13: Silence, Nature and Awe

1. Amie Gordon et al., 'The Dark Side of the Sublime: Distinguishing a Threat-Based Variant of Awe,' *Journal of Personality and Social Psychology* 113, no. 2 (2017): 310–28, https://doi.org/10.1037/pspp0000120; Joanna Pearce et al., 'What Fosters Awe-Inspiring Experiences in Nature-Based Tourism Destinations?,' *Journal of Sustainable Tourism* 25, no. 3 (2015): 362–78, https://doi.org/10.1080/09669582.2016 .1213270; Jennifer E. Stellar et al., 'Self-Transcendent Emotions and Their Social Functions: Compassion, Gratitude, and Awe Bind Us to Others through Prosociality,' *Emotional Review* 9, (June 2017), https://doi.org/10.1177/1754073916684557.

2. Dacher Keltner and Jonathan Haidt, 'Approaching Awe, a Moral, Spiritual, and Aesthetic Emotion,' *Cognition and Emotion* 17, no. 2 (2003): 297–314, https://doi .org/10.1080/02699930302297; Michelle N. Shiota et al., 'The Nature of Awe: Elicitors, Appraisals, and Effects on Self-Concept,' *Cognition and Emotion* 21, no. 5 (July 2007): 944–63, https://doi.org/10.1080/02699930600923668.

3. Keltner and Haidt, 'Approaching Awe,' 297–314; Paul K. Piff et al., 'Awe, the Small Self, and Prosocial Behavior,' *Journal of Personality and Social Psychology* 108, no. 6 (2015): 883–899, https://doi.org/10.1037/pspi0000018; Huanhuan Zhao et al.,

'Relation Between Awe and Environmentalism: The Role of Social Dominance Orientation,' *Frontiers in Psychology* 9, (December 2018), https://doi.org/10.3389/fpsyg.2018.02367.

4. Michelle N. Shiota et al., 'Positive Emotion Dispositions Differentially Associated with Big Five Personality and Attachment Style,' *The Journal of Positive Psychology* 1, no. 2 (February 2007): 61–71, https://doi.org/10.1080/17439760500510833.

5. Melanie Rudd et al., 'Awe Expands People's Perception of Time, Alters Decision Making, and Enhances Well-Being,' *Psychological Science* 23, no. 10 (August 2012), https://doi.org/10.1177/0956797612438731; Patty Van Cappellen and Vassilis Saroglou, 'Awe Activates Religious and Spiritual Feelings and Behavioral Intentions,' *Psychology of Religion and Spirituality* 4, no. 3 (2012): 223–36, https://doi.org/10.1037/a0025986.

6. Libin Jiang et al., 'Awe Weakens the Desire for Money,' *Journal of Pacific Rim Psychology* 12 (January 2018), https://doi.org/10.1017/prp.2017.27.

7. Sara B. Algoe and Jonathan Haidt, 'Witnessing Excellence in Action: The "Other-praising" Emotions of Elevation, Gratitude, and Admiration,' *The Journal of Positive Psychology* 4, no. 2 (March 2009): 105–27, https://doi.org/10.1080/17439760802650519; Edward T. Bonner and Harris L. Friedman, 'A Conceptual Clarification of the Experience of Awe: An Interpretative Phenomenological Analysis,' *The Humanistic Psychologist* 39, no. 3 (2011): 222–35, https://doi.org/10.1080/08873267.2011.593372.

8. Jennifer E. Stellar et al., 'Self-Transcendent Emotions and Their Social Functions: Compassion, Gratitude, and Awe Bind Us to Others through Prosociality,' *Emotion Review* 9, no. 3 (June 2017): 200–7, https://doi.org/10.1177/1754073916684557; Keltner and Haidt, 'Approaching Awe,' 297–314; Libin Jiang et al., 'Awe Weakens the Desire for Money,' *Journal of Pacific Rim Psychology* 12 (January 2018), https://doi.org/10.1017/prp.2017.27; Piff 'Awe, the Small Self, and Prosocial Behavior,' 883–99; Claire Prade and Vassilis Saroglou, 'Awe's Effects on Generosity and Helping,' *The Journal of Positive Psychology* 11 (January 2016): 522–30, https://doi.org/10.1080/17439760.2015.1127992; Amie Gordon et al., 'The Dark Side of the Sublime: Distinguishing a Threat-Based Variant of Awe,' *Journal of Personality and Social Psychology* 113, no. 2 (2017): 310–28, https://doi.org/10.1037/pspp0000120.

9. Jennifer E. Stellar et al., 'Self-Transcendent Emotions and Their Social Functions: Compassion, Gratitude, and Awe Bind Us to Others through Prosociality,' *Emotion Review* 9, no. 3 (June 2017): 200–7, https://doi.org/10.1177/1754073916684557.

10. Melanie Rudd et al., 'Awe Expands People's Perception of Time, Alters Decision Making, and Enhances Well-Being,' *Psychological Science* 23, no. 10 (August 2012), https://doi.org/10.1177/0956797612438731.

11. Cherisse L. Seaton and Sherry L. Beaumont, 'Pursuing the Good Life: A Short-Term Follow-up Study of the Role of Positive/Negative Emotions and

Ego-Resilience in Personal Goal Striving and Eudaimonic Well-Being,' *Motivation and Emotion* 39 (April 2015): 813–26, https://doi.org/10.1007/s11031-015-9493-y; Jiang, 'Awe Weakens the Desire for Money.'

12. Andrew J. Howell et al., 'Meaning in Nature: Meaning in Life as a Mediator of the Relationship Between Nature Connectedness and Well-Being,' *Journal of Happiness Studies* 14 (2013): 1681–96, https://doi.org/10.1007/s10902-012-9403-x.

13. Barbara L. Fredrickson and Thomas Joiner, 'Positive Emotions Trigger Upward Spirals Toward Emotional Well-Being,' *Psychological Science* 13, no. 2 (March 2002): 172–5, https://doi.org/10.1111/1467-9280.00431.

14. Ed Diener, 'Subjective Well-Being: The Science of Happiness and a Proposal for a National Index,' *American Psychologist* 55, no. 1 (2000): 34–43, https://doi.org/10.1037/0003-066X.55.1.34.

15. Sonja Lyubomirsky, 'Why Are Some People Happier than Others? The Role of Cognitive and Motivational Processes in Well-Being,' *American Psychologist* 56, no. 3 (2001): 239–49, https://doi.org/10.1037/0003-066X.56.3.239.

16. Ed Diener et al., 'Personality, Culture, and Subjective Well-Being: Emotional and Cognitive Evaluations of Life,' *Annual Review of Psychology* 54 (February 2003): 403–25, https://doi.org/10.1146/annurev.psych.54.101601.145056; Michael F. Steger, 'Meaning in Life,' in *The Oxford Handbook of Positive Psychology*, eds C. R. Snyder and Shane J. Lopez (New York, NY: Oxford University Press, 2009): 679–87, https://doi.org/10.1093/oxfordhb/9780195187243.001.0001.

17. Neal Krause and R. David Hayward, 'Awe of God, Congregational Embeddedness, and Religious Meaning in Life,' *Review of Religious Research* 57 (2015): 219–38, https://doi.org/10.1007/s13644-014-0195-9.

18. Matthew McDonald et al., 'The Nature of Peak Experience in Wilderness,' *The Humanistic Psychologist* 37, no. 4 (2009): 370–85, https://doi.org/10.1080/08873260701828912; Huanhuan Zhao et al., 'Relation Between Awe and Environmentalism: The Role of Social Dominance Orientation,' *Frontiers in Psychology* 9, (December 2018), https://doi.org/10.3389/fpsyg.2018.02367; Todd M. Thrash et al., 'Inspiration and the Promotion of Well-Being: Tests of Causality and Mediation,' *Journal of Personality and Social Psychology* 98, no. 3 (2010): 488–506, https://doi.org/10.1037/a0017906.

19. Christopher Peterson and Martin E. P. Seligman, *Character Strengths and Virtues: A Handbook and Classification*, (New York, NY: Oxford University Press, 2004).

INDEX

Page numbers followed by f refer to figures; those followed by t refer to tables.

protein in, 65, 67–68, 73t
as unprocessed food, 65, 67–68, 94, 96
red wine, 25–26
Reeves, Dan, 20–21, 23, 28
resilience, 112, 162, 162f
    in cold water immersion, 146, 148–51
    in mindfulness, 171
    in optimism, 173
resistance training, 115, 120, 124–27
    and aerobic training, 128
    belly fat reduced in, 119–20
    with body weight, 127
    exercises recommended, 125, 126t
    with lighter weights, 124
    mechanical tension in, 120, 127
    metabolic effects of, 120, 127
    minimum-effective amount, 124–26, 129
    mood improvement in, 127
    muscle damage in, 120, 124
    repetitions and sets in, 125, 126f
    rest periods in, 126t, 127
    stress in, 120, 124, 127
resting heart rate, 131
restless legs syndrome, 141
rest periods
    after exercise, compared to cold-water immersion, 148
    in high-intensity interval workouts, 121
    in resistance training, 126t, 127
rice, carbohydrates in, 77, 84, 85t, 87
ricotta, protein in, 73t
Rider and Elephant metaphor on decision making, 7–8, 17–18
Roosevelt, Franklin D., 91
rugby, Wilkinson in, 111, 112, 129–30
runners
    Holmes, 75–76, 89–90
    Radcliffe, 131–32, 143

running
    calories used in, 50
    in middle-distance events, 75
    sprint training in, 121–23
rutabaga, 85t, 86

S

saccharides, 76–77
salmon, 51t, 64
    omega-3 fats in, 101, 103
    protein in, 73t
salt in ultra-processed foods, 33, 34, 37, 40
sardines
    omega-3 fats in, 101, 103
    protein in, 73t
satellite cells, 154
saturated fats, 93–99, 102
    in animal protein, 67, 93–99
    in dark chocolate, 97
    in processed foods, 78
sauna use, 151–53
sausage, 67, 96, 101
scallops
    omega-3 fats in, 103
    protein in, 73t
Scherr, Johannes, 27
Schoenfeld, Brad, 120, 125
Schweitzer, Albert, 144
sea algae, omega-3 fats in, 103
seafood. See fish and seafood
second meal effect, 47
self-awareness
    of personality traits, 160–61
    of values, 164–66
self-talk, 166–68
    in best-self exercise, 172
    confidence building, 167–68
    negative, 16, 18, 166–67
    positive, 5, 168, 173
serotonin, 56
shaping the path, 8

ABOUT THE AUTHOR

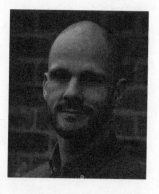

Dr Marc Bubbs, ND, MSc, CISSN, CSCS is a naturopathic doctor, performance nutrition lead for Canada Basketball and performance nutrition consultant for a portfolio of professional and Olympic athletes. Marc is the author of the best-selling book *Peak: The New Science of Athletic Performance That is Revolutionizing Sports*. Marc also hosts *The Performance Nutrition Podcast*, connecting listeners with world-leading experts in human performance and health, and regularly speaks at health, fitness and medical conferences across North America, the UK and Europe. Marc practices in both Toronto, Canada and London, England.

DrBubbs.com
The Performance Nutrition Podcast
YouTube @DrBubbs
Twitter @DrBubbs
Instagram @DrBubbs
Facebook @DrBubbs